HEALTH TELEMATICS FOR
CLINICAL GUIDELINES AND PROTOCOLS

Studies in Health Technology and Informatics

Editors

Jens Pihlkjaer Christensen, CEC DG XIII/C-AIM, Brussels
Tim De Dombal, University of Leeds
Jaap Noothoven van Goor †, ACOSTA, Brussels
Antonio Pedotti, Politecnico di Milano
Viviane Thévenin, CEC DG XII/F BIOMED-I, Brussels
Christoph Zywietz, Medizinische Hochschule Hannover

Volume 16

ISSN: 0926-9630

Health Telematics for Clinical Guidelines and Protocols

Edited by

C. Gordon

Royal Brompton Hospital NHS Trust, London

and

J.P. Christensen

European Commission, DG XIII, Brussels

1995
IOS Press

Ohmsha

Amsterdam, Oxford, Tokyo, Washington, DC

ISBN 90 5199 199 1 (IOS Press)
ISBN 4 274 90024 X C3047 (Ohmsha)

Publisher
IOS Press
Van Diemenstraat 94
1013 CN Amsterdam
Netherlands

Distributor in the UK and Ireland
IOS Press/Lavis Marketing
73 Lime Walk
Headington
Oxford OX3 7AD
England

Distributor in the USA and Canada
IOS Press, Inc.
P.O. Box 10558
Burke, VA 22009-0558
USA

Distributor in Japan
Ohmsha, Ltd.
3-1 Kanda Nishiki - Cho
Chiyoda - Ku
Tokyo 101
Japan

PRINTED IN THE NETHERLANDS

v

Contents

Preface

Guidelines and protocols for clinical practice (sometimes also termed practice policies) are receiving increasing attention from clinicians and health services as means for applying best current knowledge to maximise the quality and efficiency of delivered healthcare within the given economic constraints. This volume contains the proceedings of a Conference organized in April 1994 by the Health Telematics programme (1991-1994), the AIM programme, which forms part of the Third Framework Programme for Research and Technological Development of the Commission of the European Communities.

Earlier discussions among projects participating in this programme had confirmed the growing and widespread importance of this trend within medicine, and the widely recognised potential for healthcare telematics to facilitate the creation, use and constant improvement of clinical guidelines so as to deliver fullest benefits to patients. This observation was strongly reinforced by the results of the EPISTOL study, an accompanying action of the Health Telematics programme set up to clarify the potential impact of knowledge-based systems (KBS) for the health sector. As the chapter in this volume by Pedro Barahona reports, applications of KBS to the use of clinical guidelines were highlighted by this study as a feasible and worthwhile objective for research and development in health telematics during the next few years.

A significant number of projects within the current Health Telematics programme were found to have an active interest in this subject. Accordingly, a Conference was convened to explore the scope and needs for further work in this area. This was accomplished by means of talks by domain experts, presentations by members of all interested Health Telematics projects, and discussion of future needs and measures, including inputs to planning of the CEC 4th Framework Programme and its Health Telmatics workplan.

Twenty-two speakers contributed to the meeting, including representatives of 13 Health Telematics projects and invited experts from outside organizations (Peter C Gøtzsche, The Nordic Cochrane Centre, Denmark; Jean-Louis Renaud-Salis, French Federation of Cancer Centres; Dr Ian Purves, The Sowerby Unit for Primary Care Informatics, Newcastle). Three parallel working sessions addressed issues relating to Primary and Community Care, Secondary and Shared Care, and Guidelines and Knowledge Engineering/Methodology. Specific clinical areas of guideline use presented by speakers included: general medical practice (prevention; prescribing; chronic disease management), cancer, cardiology, neurology, gastro-enterology, rehabilitation, shared care and intensive care.

Some of the conclusions and practical recommendations which emerged from the Conference are reported in Colin Gordon's chapter below. We believe that these Proceedings form an important addition to the literature of health telematics, reflecting the range and depth of innovative talent mobilised in the current European Health Telematics programme. We hope they provide some pointers towards practical ways in which telematics can help meet the health objectives of European citizens, governments, and healthcare professionals.

Colin Gordon and Jens Pihlkjaer Christensen (Editors)

Acknowledgements

Members of the following projects in the 1991-94 AIM programme contributed presentations to the conference "Health Telematics for Clinical Guidelines and Protocols": DILEMMA, ESTEEM, GALEN, GAMES-II, IREP, ISAAC, KAVAS-2, OPADE, NUCLEUS, PROCAS, TANIT and TELEGASTRO. The Head of CEC DG XIII Health Telematics, Niels Rossing, delivered the Welcoming Address. We are grateful to Dr Rossing for his support of this Conference.

The conference programme was organised by Colin Gordon on behalf of the DILEMMA project and AIMCOM Project Line 3 (Knowledge-Based Systems), comprising the DILEMMA, ESTEEM, GALEN, GAMES-II, HELIOS-2, KAVAS-2 and OPADE projects, with additional assistance from the members of the GAMES-II, ISAAC and and PROCAS project, in conjunction with Jens P Christensen and Jennifer Delahunt (Health Telematics Central Office), who handled conference arrangements in Brussels and compiled the Draft Proceedings. The rapporteurs of the Conference working sessions were Ian Herbert, Stephen Todd and Pedro Barahona. The Select Bibliography to this volume was kindly contributed by Ian Purves.

Overviews

Health Telematics for Clinical Guidelines and Protocols
C. Gordon and J.P. Christensen (Eds.)
IOS Press, 1995

Practice guidelines and healthcare telematics: towards an alliance

Colin Gordon

Information Directorate, Royal Brompton Hospital, Sydney Street, London SW3 6NP

Abstract. This chapter reviews the motives behind the promotion, development and application of practice guidelines, defined as 'systematically developed statements to assist practitioner and patient decisions about appropriate health care for specific clinical circumstances'. It surveys the state of progress and future prospects for telematics applications in this area, and reports the action points recommended by the 1994 AIM Conference. There exists significant evidence that use of guidelines can improve healthcare process and outcome, and that computerised aids assist this effect. they may also enhance the potential uses of guidelines and protocols for audit, resource management and shared care. A standard generic model for computerised representation of guidelines as knowledge bases in a common format has been proposed and may be a key factor in future progress. The development of computerised patient records of adequate scope and quality is generally recognised as an essential condition for computer-aided guideline use. Support for development, dissemination and application of healthcare guidelines and use has emerged, notably through the AIM EPISTOL study, as a feasible and useful application area of medical knowledge-based systems. It is essential that telematics developments in this field are grounded in an understanding of the healthcare practices to which guidelines are being applied, and of the changes in practice which guideline use may entail.

1. Introduction

The USA Institute of Medicine has published the following definition of practice guidelines: "practice guidelines are 'systematically developed statements to assist practitioner and patient decisions about appropriate health care for specific clinical circumstances'" [2].

The motives and objectives of those promoting the development of clinical practice guidelines are summed up in the Institute of Medicine's statement of "Desirable Attributes of Clinical Practice Guidelines" [2]. They should, it considers, possess the following attributes:

Validity. A valid guideline is one which, when followed, leads to the outcomes projected for it. A guideline should be accompanied by a statement of the **strength of evidence** and expert judgement which support is recommendations. It should be accompanied by **estimates of the outcomes** it is expected to produce, compared with those of alternative policies, and weighed against consideration of patients' own preferences.

- **Reliability and reproducibility.** This criterion requires that different working panels, given the same guideline development method and the same evidence, should be expected to produce essentially the same guideline; and that different healthcare actors, applying the same guideline to the same case circumstances, should be expected to take the essentially the same course of action.

- **Clinical applicability.** Guidelines should define the patient population to which they apply, and they should be as broadly applicable as the evidence and expert judgement permit.
- **Clinical Flexibility.** Guidelines should explicitly identify circumstances in which their recommendations may not apply, paying particular attention to the role of patient preferences.
- **Clarity.** Guidelines should be unambiguous, precise, logically structured and easy to follow.
- **Multidisciplinary process.** All groups affected by the recommendations of a guideline should participate in its development.
- **Scheduled review**. Guidelines should state when their contents will be reviewed to take account of changing evidence or professional consensus.
- **Documentation.** Guidelines should thoroughly document by what methods, by whom, and on what evidential basis they were developed.

These criteria reflect the fact that the initiative for developing practice guidelines which has been gathering pace over the past few years forms part of a wider movement of opinion in favour of evidence-based, or "knowledge-based" medicine. The promoters and practitioners of clinical guideline development share, in this respect, a common cause with another constituency whose work and aims are described elsewhere in this volume by Peter Gotzsche. Within the past few years, this group has begun to organize a remarkable new world-wide organization, the Cochrane Collaboration, linking the work of all those engaged in the systematic review and dissemination of the results of randomised controlled trials (RCTs) in healthcare. The output of the Cochrane reviewing process will consist of a library of modules assembling validated scientific evidence on the effectiveness of specific healthcare interventions and policies. This material, along with other results of clinical and health service research, will form the essential input to the guideline development process envisaged by the Institute of Health and others as the means towards improving future healthcare practice and establishing what the British Medical Journal has termed a "knowledge-based health service".

It is clear that those engaging in the organization of systematic RCT reviewing and of guideline development share some common motives. Abundant evidence exists that best known clinical practice is not being generally applied, and that long and indefensible delays occur between the emergence of definitive evidence of the effectiveness or ineffectiveness of specific medical interventions, and corresponding changes in the actual performance of such interventions by practising clinicians. Global pressures on healthcare resources are obliging health service funders to conduct closer critical scrutiny of the appropriateness and cost-effectiveness of medical interventions. Widespread evidence has emerged of unjustifiable variations, within and between countries, in the quality of patient care, with consequences manifested in terms of unequal levels of care, unequal outcomes and avoidable mortality and morbidity. (In the UK, such evidence has been cited covering such major domains as the treatment of breast cancer, diabetes and asthma.)

The development and dissemination of clinical practice guidelines forms one policy for targeting areas of healthcare where there is clear evidence of what constitutes best practice and where there is evidence that the shortcomings of existing practice have adverse consequences and are capable of being improved. The creation of guidelines by appropriate expert and consensus bodies is, in principle, well accepted by healthcare professionals, and the dissemination of guidelines appears to form an efficient medium to carry out in-service training to inform practitioners of developments in the state of the art. Guideline dissemination (as Russell and Grimshaw report [5]) is more effective where it is linked to an explicit educational initiative; conversely, as Pritchard argues [22], technology which helps the practitioner to absorb new knowledge by applying it in the context of actual practice (so-called "hot learning") may constitute the most efficient form of education. Computer software linked to guidelines can supplement the work of the patient consultation, by providing patients with a written explanation of the course of treatment they are receiving, together with information for subsequent reference on medications, side-effects, lifestyle issues etc. Clinical guidelines or protocols, suitably tailored for local organizational circumstances, may provide an effective means to implement workable policies for improved resource management and provide better co-ordination of primary and hospital care.

One might sum up by saying that the attraction of clinical guidelines consists in certain common desired features they are perceived to offer: the provision of *rational, consistent* policies based on *explicit grounds* and *objective evidence*, including due consideration of *best resource use* and *patient preferences*.

2. Indicators.

The Conference reported in this volume is one among many recent manifestations of growing interest in the question of clinical guidelines. The Library of the British Medical Association in London is a major national reference resource for medical research; it recently reported that one third of all incoming requests for literature now come from prospective authors of clinical guidelines. Not surprisingly, the USA, as the scene of particularly intense recent efforts in health reform, has taken some early initiatives in public promotion of guideline development.
- In 1989, an Act of Congress established the Agency for Health Care Policy and Research (A.H.C.P.R.) with a remit to conduct a national programme to develop and promote practice guidelines. This programme is documented at length in the two volumes edited by Marilyn J Field and Kathleen N Lohr for the Institute of Medicine: *Clinical Practice Guidelines: Directions for a New Program*, and *Guidelines for Clinical Practice: From Development to Use*. [1,2]
- The question of methods of guideline development has been the subject of a number of key papers published around the same time by David Eddy and his collaborators which are summarised in his 1992 volume *Assessing Health Practices and Designing Practice Policies. The Explicit Approach* [3].

In Europe although no governmental initiative of similar extent has been undertaken, several important national projects have been started within the medical community.
- The Dutch College of General Practitioners has been engaged since 1988 in a programme of standards development for general practice, with major associated projects for computerised dissemination and implementation. [4]; cf. the chapters in this volume by Ten Hoopen et. al and Zanstra and Beckers [8,9]).
- In 1993, the French Federation of Cancer Centres (FNCLCC) initiated a National Cancer Standards Action, involving a nation-wide panel of oncologists in the development of agreed guidelines for cancer care.

- In 1994, the UK Royal College of General Practice created a *Guideline Skills Course* to assist developers of guidelines in primary care.

Lastly, it is significant that by 1993, Grimshaw and Russell were able to a publish a review covering a substantial existing literature of scientific trials of the use of clinical guidelines (including examples of computerised guideline implementation).[5]

Are clinical guidelines effective?

Grimshaw and Russell stated the conclusion of their review conclusions as follows: "We have identified 59 published evaluations of clinical guidelines that met defined criteria for scientific rigour... All but 4 of these studies detected significant improvements in the process of care after the introduction of guidelines and all but 2 of the 11 studies that assessed the outcome of care reported significant improvements".

What makes guideline-based quality initiatives effective?

Grimshaw and Russell went on to identify factors characterising the more successful guideline initiatives investigated in their review, in terms of the three stages of the guideline lifecycle: *development, dissemination* and *implementation*.

- **Development: User involvement in guideline development.** Grimshaw and Russell found that users most often accepted a guideline where they or their representatives had participated in its development. They were more likely to believe it had been properly developed, more likely to feel ownership of its content, and more confident of its appropriateness to their practice requirements. This finding nevertheless presents a challenge to guideline developers, since the essential literature and evidence reviewing processes which should precede guideline development are likely to be feasible only at a national or international level of organization. A possible two-stage formula to resolve this dilemma would comprise a two-stage process of centralised collation of evidence, followed by localised adaptation of evidence modules to produce guidelines tailored to local processes, populations and resources. (Cf. the discussion of these findings by Ian Purves elsewhere in this volume.[21])
- **Dissemination: Specific education intervention.** Where the dissemination of a guideline was explicitly presented as a form of in-service training, and accompanied by dedicated educational material, clinicians were more likely to read and take notice of the guideline.
- **Implementation: Patient-specific reminder at time of consultation.** Guidelines were found to be most effectively implemented when their implications for an individual patient case were identified and presented to the clinician at the time of the consultation: that is to say, when only currently relevant elements within a guideline were drawn to the clinician's attention in a live setting. A computerised system, it was found, could perform this selecting and presenting function effectively in systems where an electronic patient record allowed relevant factors to be identified automatically.

3. Uncertainties and caveats.

Rational and persuasive as the grounds for supporting the development of guidelines may be, there are several reasons for tempering any excessive optimism about their short-term practical effects.

Will they be used?

As ten Hoopen et al. report in this volume, Dutch doctors approve of the dissemination of standards but it is not clear how far they are inclined to apply them. Anecdotal evidence indicates that doctors are happiest in endorsing the use of guidelines by practitioners other than themselves: consultants approve of protocols for the guidance of junior doctors; hospital specialists are keen to see good practice disseminated to GPs; GPs approve of guidelines for use by practice nurses, but may be less willing to follow them in their own consultations. Using guidelines in medicine is sometimes felt to be demeaning, deskilling, and professionally mediocre - reactions expressed in the pejorative phrase "cookbook medicine". (A British patient, aware of the beneficial effects of Elizabeth David's writings on national cooking practices, might find other and more encouraging implications in such a turn of phrase.) Guidelines ought not to undermine the freedom of clinical judgement, unless they are given improper mandatory force. Anxieties of this kind may well linger for some time, but the view expressed by Professor Michael Peckham, Head of Research in the UK National Health Service perhaps better expresses the current trend of opinion: "it would be hard for clinicians to resist guidelines about the best way forward, if 'we have developed appropriate research information, and explained this properly'... 'differences in clinical practice that matter, will not be justifiable if there is valid data on the problem. *I am absolutely convinced that this approach will liberate clinicians.'"*[6]

Can all guidelines be successfully applied?

Although Russell and Grimshaw have assembled encouraging evidence that the use of guidelines can improve both process and outcome, and that these results are positively associated with the use of computerised aids, it is not altogether clear how far such documented successes can be reproduced, because many published guidelines, including those of the A.H.C.P.R. appear to be considerably more complex and extensive in scope than those guidelines successfully implemented in relatively simple and effective "reminder" systems such as Regenstrief and HELP [19,20]. As the guidelines to be applied become more complex, the key task of identifying the relevant patient-specific implications of a guideline at any one time is liable to become considerably more demanding.

More advanced guideline support systems, although now judged to be technically feasible with existing medical informatics and knowledge-based systems techniques, might fail in various ways to perform adequately or to gain acceptance. It appears to be feasible to implement a system capable of informing a doctor or nurse what actions a given guideline recommends in the current care of a given patient problem; it would be a more challenging to provide a system which could explain intelligently whether or why such a recommendation ought to be followed in a given case, or how the advice of different guidelines should be synthesised in a case involving multiple problems. The scale of the knowledge engineering task involved in such an undertaking should not be underestimated.

Will they be workable?

Even the more straightforward type of computer functionality, however, can only be effectively delivered on the basis of an adequate electronic patient record. This is because a guideline system will only be acceptable if it determines the part of the guideline relevant to a specific patient case, and it can only determine this by inference from the data of that case. This in turn requires, firstly that the electronic practice system is actually capable of recording patient information in an sufficiently structured and expressive format and using a standardised vocabulary, and secondly that clinicians are able and motivated to record patient data on such a system (bearing in mind that most recording must take place, if at all, during the patient consultation).

Will they be usable and worth using?

A final set of reservations are in order concerning the intrinsic value and applicability of guidelines. Much of the argument in favour of RCTs and evidence-based medicine concerns the impressive evidence of the fallibility of medical expertise and clinical judgement. The problem, with respect to guideline *value*, is that it is seldom possible to logically derive the content of a clinical guideline solely from the results of a set of reviewed RCTs: in some respects a guideline will never be more than a statement of carefully distilled opinion. Guidelines are invented, not deduced, and their creation is an art rather than a science - albeit an art in which sound methods and procedures can be learned and practised. Possibly the most that can be ensured in this respect is the use, in Eddy's term, of an explicit method such that each recommendation of a guideline is provided with an explicitly stated justification. So far as the *applicability* of guidelines is concerned, the Institute of Health's criteria, if systematically followed, would seem ensure that clinical guidelines are capable of being applied: that is, that their recommendations are clear and comprehensible *and that it is actually feasible for a practitioner to elicit and apply these recommendations at every appropriate stage within the process of care.* (Following a guideline is, after all, a means to perform a limited part, not the whole, of the activities of healthcare, and it must not impeded these other activities, especially the activity of communicating with the patient.)

At present, there is no way to guarantee that this result is achieved. For the moment, the key moral for developers of technology to support guideline use is to start by understanding (and building explicit, formal models of) the processes of care which a guideline is intended to support. Such models can, moreover, provide the best basis for a successful approach to representing the knowledge content of guidelines in a serviceable electronic format.[12,13,14]

Maxim: first understand the healthcare process.

When designing aids to the application of clinical guidelines, it is essential to thoroughly understand the processes of care which the guideline addresses and within which it is intended to be used. In fact one can go further: part of the intention of introducing new guidelines is commonly to reorganise or otherwise modify the process of care, and the simple fact of using and applying a guideline is itself likely to involve or entail some such degree of reorganization. In the current jargon, introducing guidelines involves, or is part of a process of healthcare business process re-engineering: proper consideration of the nature of that process is, as several contributors to this volume have emphasised, likely to be an essential preliminary step for designers of telematics to support guideline use.

4. Guidelines, protocols and audit.

There are, evidently, close relations between changing healthcare practice, measuring healthcare quality and conducting research into healthcare effectiveness and outcome. Use of telematics may help to draw these activities together into more effective synergy, but it is first useful to be clear about what each activity involves.

Guidelines and Protocols: What's in a Name?

The words 'guideline' and 'protocol' are, as is often remarked, widely used in inconsistent or interchangeable ways. The Institute of Medicine offers a serviceable standard definition of 'practice guideline' but does not formally define (or use) the term 'protocol'. However, the sense in which the term 'protocol' tends to be used in current discourse does embody an important and useful distinction which it is worth retaining and making explicit.

To begin with, it is broadly true that any use of the term "guideline" or "protocol" refers to an instance of one or more of the following ideal-typical categories:

- **Guidelines of best practice**, preferably derived from evidence by a recognised methodology adapted as necessary for local resources and conditions. These may cover an extended area of clinical management (e.g. chronic asthma care), or a single action in a single context (e.g. monitor for a side-effect of a prescribed drug). Compliance with guidelines is usually voluntary, though there may be some obligation to consult, or at least have access to a guideline on a given topic.
- **Protocols for carrying out an exact agreed policy (policy protocols)** for some healthcare business functions (e.g. booking a follow-up appointment or writing a discharge letter). Such protocols are not necessarily or typically addressed to guiding decision-making as such, but they can crucially affect the quality of decision-making and clinical care.
- **Protocols of a clinical trial (trial protocols)**. By definition, a successful trial demands adherence to a precisely defined protocol. A trial protocol will, like a guideline, define the required conduct of a care activity, together with added activities specific to a trial, such as randomization, procedure for informed consent, and communication between trial sites and trial coordinators.

There are several overlaps between these categories. In oncology, the protocol of a successful trial may perhaps with (minor adaptation) become the hospital's guideline for routine best practice. In oncology, again, key standardised elements of protocol (typically, those defining complex and intrinsically hazardous interventions, such as chemotherapy regimens) are equally necessary to ensure the validity of research and the safety of clinical practice. Policy protocols and best practice guidelines may be viewed as approaches from different directions (respectively bottom-up and top-down) to different ends of the same problem. Pitty et. al. thus describe, elsewhere in this volume, initiatives in a domain (cardiology) where formal practice guidelines are somewhat less widely applied than in oncology, but where telematics can help implement policy protocols to ensure basic conditions of effective care in terms of the storage and communication of patient information. [10, 11] The chapters by Wilson et. al. and Rossi-Mori et al. similarly discuss scenarios (respectively in the areas of intensive care and rehabilitation) where policy protocols are necessary to effectively coordinate the cooperative activity of multiple healthcare agents. [16,17] In general, it is likely that the final stage of adapting a centrally devised guideline to best practice for local use will involve adding to the guideline policy protocol components (such as locally agreed referral criteria or datasets, or a local practice drug formulary) reflecting local organizational factors. As Pitty et. al suggest, computerised protocols of this kind offer the potential to support real-time resource management, by implementing a global planning policy at a case-sensitive level. (They also provide the possibility of generating workload measurement and analysis data considerably superior to that of current case-mix measures).

Guidelines and audit: what's the difference?

Many of those currently engaged in developing, disseminating or applying practice guidelines have also been involved in recent years in promoting and practising the activity of clinical audit. It is worth briefly reviewing the relationship of clinical guidelines to clinical audit. The two terms denote distinct, but closely related and interdependent approaches to the improvement of healthcare quality.

In the United Kingdom, hospitals and health centres now commonly have an explicit quality policy which is implemented via organised procedures for standards setting and audit, based on health service requirements and recognised best practice methods. During the course of a year, a hospital Medical Audit Office may provide support for the conduct of (perhaps 10 or 20) major audits of aspects of hospital practice, and (perhaps 50) audit meetings reviewing specific areas of hospital practice, documented in an annual report. A hospital Quality Office may centrally maintain a library of all standards and audit tools defined and used in these activities, and provide technical assistance in creating audit standards and audit forms. It is quite likely that the majority of existing audit standards are probably addressed to topics of nursing care, but they may also cover medical practice, and some standards may in either case take the form of true clinical guidelines or protocols. Computerisation is widely recognised as a practical aid in medical audit, but is often infeasible in the absence of a computerised record of patient care.

Audit methodology commonly emphasises that its role is not to monitor the totality of clinical practice, nor to prescribe complete or optimal definitions of what is good practice. Audit typically focuses on a limited set of significant, measurable and modifiable indicators by which clinical practice in a given total set of cases or episodes can be measured against some quantitative norm. An audit standard will contain an explicit statement of the norm in question. The existence of an audit standard may be intended to consciously influence clinical conduct in individual cases, although it may not necessarily indicate what must be done in every single such case, and (in the case of standards expressed in terms of target populations and percentages) it may not be achievable by means of individual case-specific decisions. Audit is concerned, in Donabedian's classic triad, with *structure, process* and *outcome*: it measures action (process), the means of action (structure) and its consequences (outcome); though not all audit initiatives address all three at once. Clinical practice guidelines may deal with both structure and process; outcomes measured by audit (and, more formally, by clinical trial) will show whether the consequences of implementing a guideline correspond to its authors' prediction and its users' expectation (and whether use of the guideline brings actual outcomes closer to those which are being sought).

Guidelines can be used either to directly influence practice at the level of individual cases and decisions, or for (prospective and retrospective) audit. Audit tests whether and how far a standards is being followed, and can be used to measure progress over time towards fuller compliance. A guideline may be intended to cover all the key elements in the management of a certain class of problem: an audit may focus on a limited check list of critical or representative items.

Retrospective audit is intended to work through interpretation and discussion by/with the professions whose activity is being audited. The simplest and most usual outcome is that individuals whose practice is shown to fall seriously short of a target standard become aware of this and are consequently prompted and motivated to move closer to the target, perhaps helped by changes to the structure, process or resourcing of care. The "audit cycle" then moves on to verify how far these corrective measures and intention take effect as a result. However the audit cycle can also be moved on by refining or shifting the focus or methodology of the audit, either because of problems raised in collecting data or because the data collected suggests a new problem to audit. The chapter in this volume by Zanstra and Beckers describes a computer system capable of generating a variety of detailed retrospective audit reports to inform practitioners how and in what respects they have succeeded in implementing a nationally agreed practice standard.

A particularly attractive possibility, proposed by Pritchard [22], is the use of a guideline to provide **concurrent audit**, to enable a clinician to check a decision against a guideline before it is made - either though some form of (possibly computer-generated) reminder, or through some computerised watchdog or critiquing system to detect and query departures from a guideline. Concurrent audit is technically harder to implement than retrospective audit, but may provide a far more effective means of changing practice, though also more liable to be resisted because of its greater intrusiveness.

Computerised support for guideline use should (on one condition: see below) be able to generate audit data as a by-product, by providing assistance for structured data collection on specific topics. Audit data should provide one input for measuring the effectiveness of a guideline and its implementation - i.e. for checking (a) whether the guideline is modifying the process of care as intended and (b) whether the modifications have beneficial outcomes for the patient. The collection of audit data can help to show, in advance of guideline development or introduction, where or whether a guideline is needed to improve the quality of care.

One caveat to be attached to this prospect of painless audit concerns the question whether the audit indicators useful for successful practice management are in fact a subset of the data required for healthcare purposes, and which a computer system would help to record as a matter of routine. Ten Hoopen suggests, however, that experience from management systems development in other sectors indicates that this postulate may be incorrect [8].

Clinical Guidelines and Heathcare Quality

Clinical guidelines have a part to play within the repertoire of healthcare quality assurance methods. Clearly, however, they are not to be seen as the only such method. Moreover, all the processes of guideline development, dissemination and application need themselves to be subject to quality assurance. The Institute of Health's criteria for guidelines provide a basis for quality assurance standards in guideline development (although it may be an illusion to suppose that guideline development methodology will ever constitute a rigorous science). The application of clinical guidelines is in itself a modification of clinical practice, and as such forms a proper object for clinical trials (and other appropriate forms of quality assurance). Trial of this kind have indeed, as we have noted, already been conducted and reviewed. Last but not least, telematics tools to support guideline use must themselves be soundly engineered.

A considerable existing investment has been made by health services in quality measures such as audit. Additional effort towards applying practice guidelines should seek to coordinate productively with this existing work.

5. Computerised guidelines and medical artificial intelligence.

The task of providing telematics support for the use of clinical guidelines has a number of attractive features for workers in medical knowledge-based systems. There is, firstly, some evidence that a health service demand for such services exists. Secondly, some (but not all) of the key problems of medical knowledge engineering have been resolved: application knowledge base contents have already been identified and constructed by guideline developers in the form of viable, validated, bounded, task-related knowledge modules; in principle, the same guideline knowledge base should be of value to many users. Thirdly, the inferencing capabilities required of a computerised guideline system (at least for a core set of basic services) are, because of the essentially categorical character of guidelines and medical statements, relatively modest and in principle achievable (but see [23] for some problems along the way). 'Deeper' reasoning tasks for computerised systems such as adapting, explaining and combining the content of clinical guidelines are, conversely, by common consent viable and worthwhile agenda items for ongoing medical AI research.

Approaches to guideline knowledge representation.

This class of KBS applications presents, however, a number of problems. Translating even a well-constructed clinical guideline of average size into a knowledge base is a non-trivial task, notably because the implicit task context in which actions addressed by a guideline are embedded needs to be made explicit in order for the guideline knowledge structure to be properly formalised. The prospects of computerised guideline dissemination and application would be much improved if a common model for the computerised representation of guideline knowledge were to be shared across the different software platforms on which guideline-based services are delivered to clinicians. Ian Herbert's chapter in this book describes one proposal, originating from the AIM project DILEMMA, for such a shared generic protocol model. Another benefit of using such a common model would be to provide guideline authors with the possibility of easy access to computerised dissemination of their output on all available software platforms, subject only to the conversion of the guideline into a model-compliant knowledge base. Knowledge authoring tools are currently being developed which would enable guideline developers to produce their own electronic knowledge bases in such a standard format. The involvement of knowledge engineering skills in the guideline development process from an early stage would certainly enhance the prospects for successful computerization, but might also provide an aid to ensuring the logical consistency, clarity and completeness of the guidelines themselves.

The weight of opinion from within the KBS community would tend to favour adopting an approach to model-based guideline knowledge representation that uses a *declarative*, rather than a *procedural* format: that is to say, a representation which contains only the knowledge content of a guideline and does not include any specific instructions on how the knowledge should be used in some computer system to deliver advice to a user. This approach (exemplified by the DILEMMA model) seems suited to maximise the benefits of transferability and reusability of knowledge, allowing different software inference systems to make use of the same knowledge-base material, and allowing the same system to make different uses of a knowledge-base to provide different services to a user. The medical KBS community has had comparatively little experience in constructing declarative models to represent knowledge about healthcare procedures and processes, but it has proved that important elements of the problem have been addressed by work (undertaken originally for other purposes) in healthcare business modelling.

An alternative approach which deserves mention has been adopted by the developers of the Arden Syntax, a collaborative international venture aimed at developing standard-format Medical Logic Modules (MLMs). [19,20] Each module comprises, in effect, a small medical protocol, providing the basis for an advice or reminder function which can be incorporated into a variety of existing computerised medical record systems. The Arden group has, until the present, made an explicit choice in favour of a procedural representation in which the representation of knowledge is fused with the specification of a specific algorithmic function for an advice/reminder system. This approach (somewhat similar to that of systems successfully introduced in UK general practice systems, such as the SOPHIE tool of AAH Meditel System 5, and the 'template' function of the EMIS system) has proved serviceable for developing some initial guideline facilities, but those with experience of this approach are also aware of its probable limits.

The benefits of common (or mutually convertible) medical knowledge representation methods have of course been under discussion for some time in other KBS application contexts. In the context of computerising clinical guidelines, these benefits are so obvious that movement towards an agreed standard is particularly urgent. The 1991-94 AIM programme has probably helped to increase momentum towards such consensus in Europe.

At the same time, discussion of this subject has thrown even greater emphasis on the need to achieve common and adequate standards for the functionality, data architecture and terminology handling capabilities of the electronic patient record. As several authors in the present volume rightly emphasise, the successful provision of telematics to support clinical guideline use is almost totally dependant on an adequate electronic patient record, and indeed places certain new demands on the functionality of such a record (particularly in terms of support for care planning).

Towards an alliance.

Pedro Barahona's chapter in this book describes how the AIM programme's EPISTOL study addressed the prospects for work on computerized guidelines in terms of the prospects for successful work in medical knowledge-based systems. [15] The conclusions of EPISTOL on this subject can be seen as either representing a prudent pragmatic realignment in response of pressure from funding programmes such as AIM, or as a deeper paradigm shift in the way the European medical AI community seeks to define goals for itself which allow its capabilities to be brought to bear on real user requirements. Perhaps both interpretations are correct. The key realignment which has been taking place might be called the shift from evaluation to value. Most medical expert systems, even those with objectively proven high problem-solving performance, have been rejected by users or, when accepted, have proved difficult to transplant outside their environment of origin. The industrially successful exceptions to this rule, such as the systems for interpreting ECGs, are, as Barahona remarks, precisely exceptions which prove the rule. Supporting clinical practice guidelines, on the other hand, is a task for the KBS community which, though perhaps somewhat less gratifying (at least at first sight) in pure research terms, means supporting objectives formulated from within the clinical user community *and which that community itself judges to be of value*. Of course the contribution of technology as an instrument of this kind of healthcare policy will require specific, objective evaluation: but what will be evaluated here will be, precisely, the ability of the technology to realise objectives which the user community has already set for itself. The health telematics community thus has the possibility of forming a productive alliance with a constituency of change agents working within the user community. In the context of prospective activity in the Fourth Framework this promises a sound basis for meeting the European Commission's requirement to move away from *'technology push'* into the direction of *'user-driven'* applications.

An approach by the telematics community which is more closely focused on the everyday concerns of clinical practice is perhaps more likely to contribute to overcoming the barrier which - as contributors to this volume have stressed - continues to marginalise the potential use of most medical KBS, namely the widespread lack of an adequate, well-structured computerised medical record. The essential role of what have hitherto been termed knowledge-based decision support systems, and might now perhaps better be called *practice and policy support systems*, is likely to lie in underpinning and enhancing the full functionality of the electronic record as an active tool for the planned management of care. [18]

6. Messages

From the preceding discussions, a few key messages are worth briefly restating.

- Patient-specific computerised reminders to clinicians have been shown to be an effective way to promote the use of practice guidelines. This requires an adequate electronic patient record. Such clinical aids can provide new tools for healthcare quality and efficiency: "concurrent audit" of clinical decisions, and "real-time resource management" enabling policies to be applied on a case-sensitive level.

  There are, however, significant issues in linking computerized guidelines to the patient record, both in relation to terminology and to database semantics and architecture. Attention is especially needed to the functional requirements on patient records to support care planning and act management. The current AIM programme has shown encouraging movement towards consensus on how these requirements are to be delivered. [7]

  Extensive introduction of guidelines involves changes in clinical working practice. These aspects must be thoroughly considered in the design of usable and acceptable guideline-based decision support tools.

- Assisting the application of practice guidelines is a useful and feasible objective for knowledge-based systems development in heath telematics. A key objective for KBS work in the area is a common formal approach to computerized representation of guideline knowledge, enabling wide dissemination and transferability of knowledge bases. Knowledge engineering expertise can also be applied to help produce clear, consistent standards of expression in the initial definition of guidelines by authoring groups. Some further R&D work is justified on deeper reasoning issues which would be involved in designing more advanced aids to clinical guideline use.

7. Health Telematics for Clinical Guidelines and Protocols: conclusions of the Conference.

The April 1994 conference of the Health telematics programme whose proceedings make up the present volume demonstrated not only the strength of interest in the domain but considerable agreement on the steps needed for its further progress.

The reports from the parallel working groups, together with the final plenary discussion, indicated a large measure of consensus on:

- the growing importance of clinical guidelines within healthcare;
- their potential as a basis for achieving improvements in European healthcare quality and efficiency;
- the important role for health telematics in facilitating such improvements, through computerised assistance in guideline development, dissemination and use.

Support was expressed for a significant emphasis being placed on this area in forthcoming health telematics activities within the 4th Framework programme. In addition, support was indicated for a number of specific actions to promote development in this area (the formulation of these action points was carried out by a follow-up working session of AIMCOM Project Line 3, comprising representatives of the DILEMMA, ESTEEM, GALEN, GAMES-II, HELIOS-II, KAVAS-2 and OPADE projects). The specific recommendations made are shown below.

Recommended Actions: Health Telematics and Clinical Guidelines in the 4th Framework.

1. Investigation of the healthcare business organization and re-engineering implications of embedding computer-aided guideline use in clinical practice.
2. Inclusion of guideline support in infrastructure provision requirements for health telematics, in terms of:
- *the electronic patient record;*
- *medical terminologies and coding systems;*
- *knowledge and data communications.*

3. Action to establish consensus on guideline knowledge representation methods and models, with the objective of preparing subsequent standards proposals in this field.
4. Organized collaboration between healthcare telematics and clinical communities on guideline development and dissemination methods, including links with:
- *Cochrane Collaborations;*
- *Guideline authoring bodies;*
- *Clinical professions.*

5. A programme of clinical trials of computerized guidelines, within the context of an overall healthcare telematics quality methodology, and of a total quality management approach to healthcare delivery.

References

[1]   Institute of Medicine (M. J. Field and K. N Lohr Eds.) Clinical Practice Guidelines. Directions for a New Program National Academy Press, Washington DC 1990

[2]   Institute of Medicine (M. J. Field and K. N. Lohr Eds.) Guidelines for Clinical Practice. From Development to Use. National Academy Press, Washington DC 1992

[3] D. M Eddy. Assessing Health Practices and Designing Practice Policies. The Explicit Approach American College of Physicians, Philadelphia 1992.

[4] R. Grol. National standard setting for quality of care in general practice: attitudes of general practitioners and response to a set of standards. BJGP, 40:361-364, 1990.

[5] J. M. Grimshaw, I. T. Russell, "Effect of clinical guidelines on medical practice: a systematic review of rigorous evaluations" (Lancet 1993, Vol 342342 27 Nov 1993 p 1317-1322).

[6] Cited in The Independent, London 1993.

[7] P. Nicklin and B. Frandji. Act Management and Clinical Guidelines.

[8] A.J. ten Hoopen, D.A. Boon, J. Nutma and P.F. de Vries Robbé. Primary Care Guidelines from an organizational point of view.

[9] P.E. Zanstra, W.P.A. Beckers. Computerized Assessment with Primary Care Guidelines in the Netherlands.

[10] D.L. Pitty, P. Reeves, A. Rickards. Protocol-Directed Shared Care in Cardiology. In: Health Telematics for Clinical Guidelines and Protocols. C. Gordon and J.P. Christensen (Eds.), IOS Press,1994

[11] D. L Pitty, P I. Reeves. Developing Decision Support Systems: A Change in Emphasis. Proceedings of 12th International Congress of the European Federation for medical Informatics, Lisbon, Portugal, 1994 42-45.

[12] C. Gordon, S. I. Herbert, A. Jackson-Smale. Care Protocols and Healthcare Informatics. Technology and Informatics (**10**) Artificial Intelligence in Medicine, IOS Press, 1993, 289-309

[13] S I Herbert. Informatics for Care Protocols and Guidelines: Towards a European Knowledge Model. In: Health Telematics for Clinical Guidelines and Protocols. C. Gordon and J.P. Christensen (Eds.), IOS Press,1994

[14] S I Herbert, C Gordon, A Jackson-Smale, J-L. Renaud-Salis. Protocols for Clinical Care. Proceedings of 12th International Congress of the European Federation for medical Informatics, Lisbon, Portugal, 1994 30-35

[15] P. Barahona. Guideline Based Care: The Challenge for Knowledge Based Decision Support. In: Health Telematics for Clinical Guidelines and Protocols. C. Gordon and J.P. Christensen (Eds.), IOS Press,1994

[16] A. Rossi Mori, M. De Simone, C. Lalle, F.L. Ricci. A model for the structured description of healthcare activities and related data.

[17] A J Wilson, C L Bowes and J Holland. Telematics and Protocols of Care in Critical Care Environments. In: Health Telematics for Clinical Guidelines and Protocols. C. Gordon and J.P. Christensen (Eds.), IOS Press,1994

[18] J.-L. Renaud-Salis. Distributed Clinical Management Information Systems: an Enabling Technology for Future Health Programmes.

[19] O. Wigertz, N Shahsavar, P Bågenholm, H. Åhlfeldt, H. Gill. Data-driven Medical Knowledge-Based Systems Based On Arden Syntax. In P. Barahona and J. Christensen (eds.), Knowledge and Decision in Health Telematics, IOS Press, 1994.

[20] G Hripcsak, P Ludemann, T. A. Pryor, O. Wigertz, P. Clayton. Rationale for the Arden Syntax. Computers and Biomedical Research 27, 291-324, 1994.

[21] I. Purves. Computerised Guidelines In Primary Health Care:Reflections And Implications. In: Health Telematics for Clinical Guidelines and Protocols. C. Gordon and J.P. Christensen (Eds.), IOS Press,1994

[22] P.M.M. Pritchard. Can decision making be improved? Postgraduate education for general practice. 2: 4-6, 1991.

[23] A. Glowinski. Integrating guidelines and the clinical record: the role of semantically constrained terminologies. In: Health Telematics for Clinical Guidelines and Protocols. C. Gordon and J.P. Christensen (Eds.), IOS Press,1994

Clinical practice should reflect clinical science

Peter C. Gøtzsche

Director, Nordic Cochrane Centre. Research and Development Secretariat, Rigshospitalet, Blegdamsvej 9, 2100 København Ø, Denmark

Abstract. The Cochrane Collaboration was set up in 1992 as a world-wide network for creating and disseminating systematic reviews of randomised controlled trials (RCTs) in healthcare. Systematic reviewing of RCTs is an essential stage, prior to the creation and dissemination of clinical guidelines, in the practice of evidence-based medicine. This paper is intended to provide the health telematics community with an introduction to the motives, aims and activities of the Cochrane Collaboration.

It is unreasonable to expect people such as clinicians, policy makers or patients who want reliable information about the effects of health care to unearth all the relevant evidence from reports of original research. These are far too numerous and too dispersed to be of practical value. Reviews of research thus occupy a key position in the chain which links research with clinical practice.

It is often surprisingly difficult, however, to achieve reliable retrieval and synthesis of original research results. Literature search, e.g. on MEDLINE, often identifies only half the relevant reports. Further, the quality of the research literature leaves much to be desired. In a review of reviews it was estimated that only 6% of the literature published after 1970 is scientifically sound [1]. The problems encountered relate to all stages of the research process, from design, execution, and not least to analysis and interpretation of the results [2].

Like other types of retrospective research, the science of reviewing research should be performed with great care to avoid biases and personal prejudices to influence the process. Those preparing reviews have only rarely worked systematically, however [3]. Usually, they have not written formal protocols or have searched systematically for all studies likely to provide unbiased information - in particular, randomized clinical trials (RCTs, ie trials in which patients are assigned to two or more treatments at random). Most reviewers have not taken steps to control biases and random errors during the process of selecting and analysing the studies they include in their reviews. This may explain why recommendations made by specialists sometimes are more influenced by the specialty to which they belong, rather than by the scientific evidence [4].

Because scientific principles have not generally guided reviews of research evidence, useless and even harmful forms of health care have not been distinguished efficiently from useful forms of care. Further, proposals for appropriate research have not been distinguished efficiently from proposals for inappropriate, or redundant, research. For example, more than 100 trials of antibiotic prophylaxis for caesarian sections have been conducted with an untreated control group during the twenty years in which it has been known that prophylaxis is effective in preventing serious wound infections.

Fifteen years ago, this unfortunate state of affairs made Archie Cochrane, a distinguished epidemiologist, write [5]:

"It is surely a great criticism of our profession that we have not organised a critical summary, by specialty or subspecialty, adapted periodically, of all relevant randomised controlled trials."

The first specialty to which Cochrane's approach was applied was care during pregnancy and childbirth - an area which he had singled out as being exceptionally poorly grounded in good evidence. Several hundred systematic reviews of primary studies were prepared through an international collaborative effort coordinated by Dr Iain Chalmers at the National Perinatal Epidemiology Unit in Oxford. As new evidence became available, these reviews were kept up to date and published electronically [6]. The reviews, which also appeared in paper editions [7, 8], were very well received by professionals, managers, purchasers and - perhaps most importantly of all - people using the health services.

Cochrane appreciated these developments. In 1987, the year before he died, he referred to the systematic review of RCTs of care during pregnancy and childbirth as "a real milestone in the history of randomized trials and in the evaluation of care", and suggested that other specialties should copy the methods used.

Problems in evaluating the research literature

Publication bias, i.e. the greater likelihood of publishing the results when they are positive than when they are negative, distorts our perception of the efficacy of treatments. In a review of 246 cancer trials, there was no difference, on average, between new treatments and control treatments, in trials which had included more than 100 patients [9]. In the

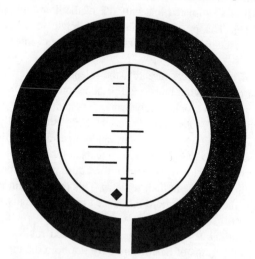

Figure 1. The Cochrane Collaboration logo illustrates a systematic review af data from seven randomized controlled trials. Each horizontal line represents the result of one trial: the shorter the line, the more certain the result. The position of the summary result, the diamond, to the left of the vertical line indicates that the treatment studied is beneficial.

smaller trials, however, the new treatments were reported to have 20-30% better survival than the control treatments. The non-randomized trials reported even greater survival benefits over control treatments, with survival ratios between 1.4 and 1.9 (increasing with decreasing sample size). This illustrates how unreliable small trials and non-randomized trials may be.

Case-control studies are not randomized and should therefore be interpreted with great caution. For example, in a study of the possible relation between induced abortion and later development of breast cancer, the difference between the reported odds ratio and the true odds ratio was 50% [10]. Although the interviewer was well trained, several of the women in the control group had failed to report that they had had an induced abortion. Fortunately, their information could be cross-checked in an abortion registry, and the error be corrected, but this is rarely the case.

Large biases have also been demonstrated when historical control groups have been used in comparisons with new treatments [11]. Technology assessment should therefore rely on randomized controlled trials whenever possible.

Expert opinion

Expert opinion is an important link between research and practice. Methodological research has shown, however, that it is rather risky to trust expert advice.

Experts tend to have strong opinions, and more so, the longer they have worked in a medical specialty. In a study in which experts were asked to judge the overall scientific quality of 36 review articles, the experts had the poorest agreement among themselves. Research assistants, physicians and methodologists agreed more [12].

Experts do not agree about effectiveness and they are often not explicit and rigorous when they state their views. For example, in two reviews of the management of bleeding oesophageal varices, which were published in the spring of 1994 in *The Lancet* and in the *British Medical Journal*, respectively, it was claimed that two different treatments could control bleeding in 90% and 95% of the cases, respectively. Such information is misleading, since bleeding often stops spontaneously; thus, the bleeding was "controlled" in 83% of those patients who were treated with placebo in a randomized trial [13].

Finally, experts do not agree with the scientific evidence. It took many years after the evidence was available, before streptokinase was recommended for routine use in acute myocardial infarction. Even after four meta-analyses had been published, several medical textbooks and review articles still did not recommend it for routine use [14]. Conversely, although all randomized trials of routine use of lidocaine indicated that it was harmful, this drug was recommended in a large number of textbooks and review articles [14]. Perhaps this discrepancy may be explained by the different clinical impression which may be experienced with the two treatments. Streptokinase may result in an occasional fatal bleeding which may have contributed to the delay in the routine use of the treatment. Lidocaine, on the other hand, can normalize certain dangerous arrhythmias and it may be difficult for the clinician to believe that the treatment can be dangerous when it normalizes the ECG. This example shows that reliance on clinical experience can be quite dangerous for the patients.

Perhaps misguided clinical logic is the reason why surveillance of high risk pregnancies with fetal cardiotocography is still widely used, despite evidence from a systematic review of RCTs that it is harmful [6]. It seems to be intuitively right to survey "just in case".

However, surveillance can lead to less rigorous clinical examination, because of undue reliance on the electronic equipment; or, conversely, since the risk of false positive alarms increases when surveillance is used, some women may be subjected to a caesarian section who would better have been left alone.

The Cochrane Collaboration

The Cochrane Collaboration was launched at the end of 1992. It is a scientific research association, supported by institu-tions and individuals in many countries.

The aims of the Cochrane Collaboration are to prepare and maintain systematic reviews of RCTs of the effects of health care, and of other evidence when appropriate, and to make this information readily available to decision-makers at all levels of health care systems. In pursuing its aims, the Cochrane Collaboration is guided by six principles: collaboration, building on people's existing enthusiasm and interests, minimizing duplication of effort, avoidance of bias, keeping up to date, and ensuring access.

The shared will to collaborate is a precondition for meeting the Collaboration's aims for two main reasons.

First, no single country has sufficient resources to sift through the daunting piles of accumulated evidence about the effects of health care which await synthesis in systematic, up-to-date reviews. Individuals with the skills and commitment required to undertake this kind of work are in short supply. Efficient international coordination is therefore important. Currently, scarce resources are being wasted because agencies in different countries or within the same country are commissioning reviews of the same evidence, without first assessing whether a relevant systematic review is already available or has been commissioned by another body.

Second, collaboration is essential, since any attempt by individuals, groups of individuals, institutions, or nations to dominate the activities of the Collaboration would have the very serious practical consequence of alienating people who could make important contributions.

The key to the success of the Collaboration is to harness the enthusiasm and energy that researchers already devote to keeping up to date in their particular areas of interest, and to provide the support they need to prepare and maintain systematic reviews. Those without such prior motivation, however, have to consider carefully the implications of committing themselves to the extent expected. The time required to prepare valid reviews is usually grossly underestimated.

Collaborative review groups

The front line contributors to the Collaboration are the reviewers. Each reviewer is a member of a collaborative review group, which consists of individuals sharing an interest in a particular topic (stroke, for example). Members of the review group seek funding from whichever sources they consider appropriate. Each collaborative review group is coordinated by an editorial team which is responsible for assembling an edited module of the reviews for incorporation in and then dissemination through the *Cochrane Database of Systematic Reviews*. In addition, the team may select reviews for compilation in one or more specialized databases. Members of the review groups may also use their electronically

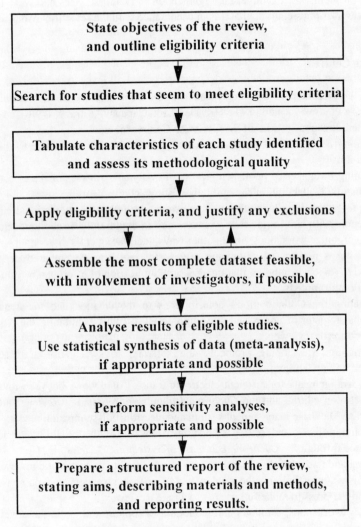

Figure 2. What is a systematic review?

published reviews as a basis for preparing printed articles and books. Although most collaborative review groups focus on health problems - breast cancer, for example - the Collaboration addresses other dimensions of interest through **field coordination**. A **field** may refer to a category of health service consumers (children, for example), a group of health professionals (intensivists, for example) a setting for health care (such as less developed countries), or a class of interventions (physical therapies, for instance). Some collaborative review groups deal with **management problems** that are common to a range of health problems, for example, the organization of health services and ways to influence the behaviour of physicians so that it is in accordance with the scientific evidence.

Cochrane Centres

Cochrane centres help to coordinate and support the Cochrane Collaboration. There are currently six centres, located in The UK, Denmark, Canada, Australia, USA, and Italy.

The shared responsibilities of the Cochrane Centres include:
• maintaining a directory of people contributing or wishing to contribute to the Cochrane Collaboration;
• maintaining a register of published reports of systematic reviews of the effects of health care, so that the Collaboration can build on existing achievements;
• helping to establish collaborative review groups, by fostering international collaboration among people with similar interests, participating in exploratory discussions and meetings, helping to organize workshops, and in other ways, facilitating collaboration;
• maintaining a register of systematic reviews currently being prepared or planned by collaborative review groups, so that unnecessary duplication of effort can be minimised and collaboration promoted;
• coordinating the Collaboration's contributions to the creation and maintenance of an international register of completed and ongoing RCTs, thus facilitating the first phase of data collection for reviewers;
• preparing and developing protocols and software to systematise and facilitate the preparation and updating of systematic reviews;
• making arrangements for efficient electronic transfer of reviews between reviewers and editors; between editors and the *Cochrane Database of Systematic Reviews*; and between the Cochrane Database management system and electronic dissemination media;
• developing policies and setting standards to maximize the reliability of information disseminated through the *Cochrane Database of Systematic Reviews*
• promoting and undertaking research to improve the quality of systematic reviews;
• exploring ways of helping the public, health service providers and purchasers, policy makers and the press to make full use of Cochrane Reviews;
• organising workshops, seminars and Colloquia to support and guide the development of the Collaboration;
• undertaking some task of service to the entire Collaboration.

Collaboration with the National Library of Medicine

The US National Library of Medicine has introduced a new publication type, *CONTROLLED-CLINICAL-TRIAL*, based on the Collaboration's definitions. This will be used for reports of controlled trials that may have been randomized or in which some quasi-random method of allocation was used. Any trials identified through the work of the Collaboration, for example, by systematically hand searching journals back to 1950, will be made accessible through MEDLINE, even if the reports have been published in journals not indexed for MEDLINE. A database of hand searched journals with contact details of the searchers has been developed to assist in this work. The criteria adopted by the Collaboration have also prompted Elsevier to adopt new methodological terms for coding controlled trials included in EMBASE.

Dissemination of systematic reviews

The guiding principles for dissemination are:
- to obtain the widest possible distribution and accessibility at reasonable price
- to maintain the integrity of the individual reviews
- to give credit where credit is due - to reviewers, editors and funders

All of the reviews prepared within the Collaboration have a standard format consisting of:
- a cover sheet, giving the title and citation details of the review; the names, addresses and other contact details, both of the reviewer(s) and of the editorial team responsible for the collaborative review group to which the reviewer(s) belong(s); and the sources of support for preparing and updating the review
- a structured report of the review, consisting of background information, the objective, the materials and methods used, the results of the review, discussion and conclusions about implications for practice and research
- full citations of reports of studies incorporated in the review, and of reports that were potentially eligible, but were excluded (with reasons for the exclusions)
- tabulation of the characteristics of the trials, with information relevant to an assessment of the methodological quality
- tabulation of the results of the review, with statistical syntheses (meta-analyses), when these were both possible and appropriate.

Because of the obvious advantages of electronic publication for systematic reviews which require maintenance as new evidence emerges and as mistakes are discovered, *The Cochrane Database of Systematic Reviews* will be disseminated online via Internet, on CD-ROM and on floppy disk. Successive versions of a review and valid criticisms will be archived electronically. Complementary arrangements will be needed to ensure that other publication forms that use Cochrane reviews are aware of substantive updates, e.g. as letters to the Editor.

The preparation of software for interrogating and displaying the reviews is not the direct responsibility of the Collaboration, but of publishers and others (for example, the Information Management Group of the UK National Health Service Management Executive). Such software is already under development. Searches will be possible both as free text and as indexed terms (MeSH).

Reviews contained in the main database are being compiled for dissemination as specialised databases on floppy disk (for example, as part of the series *Cochrane Updates on Disk*). The prototype - *The Cochrane Pregnancy & Childbirth Database* - was released in May 1993; it is updated semiannually. Compilers of specialized databases ensure that the editorial offices of each of the collaborative review groups whose reviews have been used receive copies of the published compilation on disk.

Publication of Cochrane Reviews on paper is encouraged. Concurrent electronic and paper publication has been made possible by agreements between the Cochrane Collaboration and the *British Medical Journal*, the *Lancet,* and other journals. If a print journal accepts a Cochrane review for publication, it will be modified to reflect the requirements of the journal concerned.

Communication within and outside the Cochrane Collaboration

Internet is one of the most important means of communication within the Collaboration. The electronic part of the Collaboration's work is constantly developing, in form as well as magnitude. Computer scientists are already doing important work at most of the Cochrane Centres. To be able to join progress efficiently and to serve collaborating institutions efficiently, more permanent professional assistance and guidance is necessary. The computer scientists will assist to develop data query and retrieval systems, systems for statistical analysis and display functions, report generation facilities, and data transfer and communication facilities. The computer scientists will also assist in training programmes, will provide daily technical support, and will participate actively in development work for the Collaboration so that optimal use can be made of the *Cochrane Database of Systematic Reviews* and of other databases created by the Collaboration. A collaborative network of computer scientists, working in different countries, seems to be the best way to secure that both general and local needs will be addressed in this development work.

References

[1]   Williamson JW, Goldschmidt PG, Colton T. The quality of medical literature: an analysis of validation assessments. In: Bailar III JC, Mosteller F, eds. Medical uses of statistics. Waltham: NEJM Books, 1986.

[2]   Gøtzsche PC. Bias in double-blind trials [thesis]. Dan Med Bull 1990; 37: 329-36.

[3]   Mulrow CD. The medical review article: state of the science. Ann Intern Med 1987; 104: 485-8.

[4]   Chalmers TC, Frank CS, Reitman D. Minimizing the three stages of publication bias. JAMA 1990; 263: 1392-5.

[5]   Cochrane AL. 1931-1971: a critical review, with particular reference to the medical profession. In: Medicine for the year 2000. London: Office of Health Economics, 1979: 1-11.

[6]   Cochrane Pregnancy and Childbirth Database. [Derived from the Cochrane Database of Systematic Reviews]. Published through Cochrane Updates on Disk. Oxford: Update Software, 1993, Disk Issue 1.

[7]   Chalmers I, Enkin M, Keirse MJNC, eds. Effective care in pregnancy and childbirth. Oxford: Oxford University Press, 1989.

[8]   Enkin M, Keirse MJNC, Chalmers I, eds. A guide to effective care in pregnancy and childbirth. Oxford: Oxford University Press, 1989.

[9]   Berlin JA, Begg CB, Louis TA. An assessment of publication bias using a sample of published clinical trials. J Am Stat Assoc 1989; 84: 381-392.

[10] Lindefors-Harris B-M, Eklund G, Adami H-O, Meirik O. Response bias in a case-control study: analysis utilizing comparative data concerning legal abortions from two independent Swedish studies. Am J Epidemiol 1991;134:1003-8.

[11] Sacks H, Chalmers TC, Smith H. Randomized versus historical controls for clinical trials. Am J Med 1982; 72: 233-40.

[12] Oxman AD, Guyatt GH. The science of reviewing research. In: Warren KS, Mosteller F, eds. Doing more good than harm. Ann NY Acad Sci 1993; 703: 125-33.

[13] Valenzuela JE, Schubert T, Fogel MR, Strong RM, Levine J, Mills PR, et al. A multicenter, randomized, double-blind trial of somatostatin in the management of acute hemorrhage from esophageal varices. Hepatology 1989; 10: 958-61.

[14] Antman EM, Lau J, Kupelnick B, Mosteller F, Chalmers TC. A comparison of results of meta-analyses of randomized control trials and recommendations of clinical experts: treatments for myocardial infarction. JAMA 1992; 268: 240-8.

Informatics for Care Protocols and Guidelines:Towards a European Knowledge Model

S. I. Herbert

NHS Information Management Centre, 15 Frederick Road, Birmingham B15 1JD, UK

Abstract. The DILEMMA Generic Protocol Model (DGPM) is a trans-national ontology of clinical protocols designed using a blend of logic engineering and business modelling techniques, and developed as part of the AIM programme's DILEMMA project. It allows the declarative representation of clinical activities and the knowledge associated with them. It is being used to represent protocols of all sorts - including standards and guidelines - for use in acute, primary, home and shared care. Central to the model are the states that protocol-derived actions can assume, and the statements that must be true before transitions between those states can be proposed. Proposed transitions may then be scrutinised by clinicians[1], patients and carers, and approved or rejected. This approach enables the model to handle anticipated exception situations, as well as more normal protocol selection and application. Links to multi-media material are being investigated, to enable users to examine the evidence upon which protocols are based, and to provide decision support where deterministic reasoning is not readily available. The model is being discussed with other AIM projects, with a view to developing a European consensus, and generating a version of the model for submission to CEN TC251 as a European pre-normative standard

1 Introduction

The AIM DILEMMA project is concerned with using information technology for decision support in acute oncology care, shared oncology care and primary care. Providing facilities to build and use protocols is a major component of our overall goal. To do this requires an ontology that can represent the contents of care protocols. The DILEMMA Generic Protocol Model (DGPM) contains such an ontology. This paper offers an overview of the model as of October 1994, with emphasis on its use for clinical purposes rather than resource management. Where possible, it uses simplified examples based on a protocol used by one of the DILEMMA partners to treat breast cancer. The equally essential and concomitant DILEMMA work on a protocol authoring tool, a protocol task manager, an electronic patient record design that supports protocol use and temporal qualification is mentioned only in passing. They are described fully in other DILEMMA material, although figure 1 gives a synopsis of the top-level software architecture employed.

---

[1] The term 'clinician' is used in this paper to refer to any healthcare professional, not only a doctor.

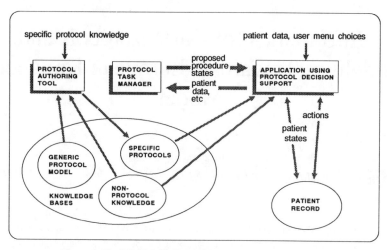

Figure 1 The DILEMMA Generic Protocol Model in Context

2 Developing the DILEMMA Generic Protocol Model

The DGPM has been developed iteratively, the current product being version 2.1. As DILEMMA partners used each version, they informed the model builders of outstanding problems and requirements. These were logged, and - where possible - were resolved in the following version.   So besides the model[1] and a companion glossary[2], there is a record[3] of all the problems and requirements encountered during development, their status and - if they were resolved - how this was done. The model is still evolving, particularly in the areas concerned with resource management, the integration of hypermedia resources and temporal qualification. The technical approach to the modelling uses Logic Engineering[4] and Business Modelling[5], and more information is available in previous papers about the DGPM[6,7]

Logic Engineering draws together the concepts of declarative programming, deductive databases and symbolic decision procedures, with a clean separation between domain knowledge and inference rules.   In the Oxford System of Medicine project [8], this approach was used to design a decision support system for primary care. In the Bordeaux Oncology Support System (BOSS), the same approach was employed in the design of a first prototype for protocol-based decision support, drawing on the valuable experience gained in the same field by the ONCOCIN project [9,10].

The Common Basic Specification (CBS) - developed by the UK National Health Service [11] - is a business model of the process of providing health care, and provides an overall framework for defining the informatics needs of clinical activities. It consists of a highly generic business activity hierarchy, the data flows entailed by those activities and a model of the data entity types involved in the dataflows.   The CBS models all aspects of 'maintaining and improving the health of a population', but DILEMMA has made particular use of the clinical view of the CBS provided by the COSMOS project [12].

3 Some essential definitions

3.1 Protocol

A protocol is a means of achieving a goal relevant to a specific *focus*, e.g. 'treat stage 1 breast cancer'. It is a template to be applied to a particular type of situation, typically a patient problem, in order to generate a plan for dealing with that situation. The description must define the protocol's focus, its *intention* vis-à-vis the focus, the *type(s) of action* required and their *sequencing*. It may cover the anticipated *outcome(s)* and *resources needed*.

A protocol may be a *standard* - i.e. describe explicitly the conditions under which all constituent actions should be performed, including those only relevant under certain circumstances - or a *guideline*, where the clinician's actions are constrained but not prescribed, and he or she must make significant decisions. A protocol may be used to *propose the care* to be provided in a particular case, to *critique the clinician's proposals for care* or to *critique the clinician's provision of care*, i.e. to carry out retrospective audit.

3.2 Protocol implementation

A protocol is *implemented* when a user applies it, or considers applying it, to a particular instance of the focus that it was designed to deal with. Protocol 'FB01' would be said to be implemented if it were deemed suitable for treating the breast cancer of Mrs Alice Springs diagnosed in June 1994.

3.3 Subject

- the object that a protocol is intended to change, risks changing or is designed to observe. In healthcare delivery it is usually a patient, but other possible subjects include a group of people, an ECG recording, a sample or an organ for transplantation.

3.4 Subject characteristic type

- something which may be observed about a subject. For a patient this might be a blood pressure, a diagnosis of measles or the presence of a stage 1 malignant breast tumour. Some characteristic types are only observable in certain types of subject: for example a blood pressure cannot be observed in a plant or a blood sample. A subject characteristic usually forms the focus for a protocol.

3.5 Agent

- an object that has the power to act, i.e. to change the state of a subject or to observe it. When planning and providing healthcare this usually means a clinician, a patient or a non-professional carer, although it could in future also include a robot.

3.6 Action

- instances of *action types*, i.e. task(s) to be performed in the real world that involve a particular subject, e.g. 'admit Mrs Springs as an inpatient to Rosycheeks ward, Wye Hospital on 21/8/93'. An action typically has a life cycle that includes being authorised,

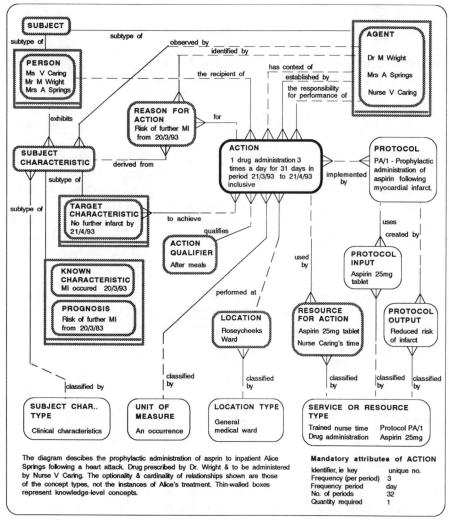

Figure 2 An instanced model of ACTION and the knowledge commonly associated with it

scheduled, started and completed; exceptionally it may be cancelled or abandoned. Figure 2 shows the information commonly associated with an action, plus examples.

3.7 Procedure

- a kind of action resulting from the implementation of a protocol. It is distinguished solely by the relationship it has to a protocol. Note that a single action can represent two protocols: if taking a blood pressure forms part of protocols for hypertension management and ante natal care being applied to the same patient, and the observations are required at about the same time, a clinician is likely to make a single observation that serves both purposes. A protocol for an iterated action will generate one procedure per iteration. A procedure may be to enable or plan care, not just provide it, so that the action - e.g. make a referral, request a test, book a clinic appointment - may not be of a type normally considered a clinical action.

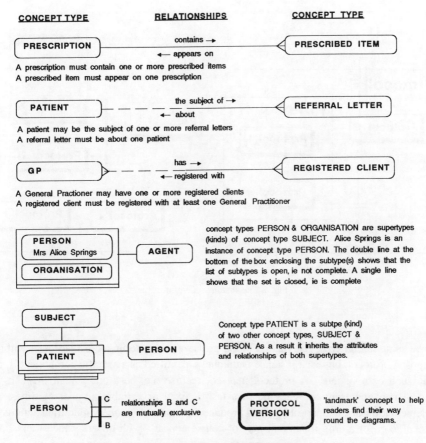

Fig 3 Key for conceptual model diagrams

4 Representing the static elements of protocol knowledge

4.1 The anatomy of a protocol

Figure 4 depicts the anatomy of an imaginary protocol, and shows the structural concepts that the DGPM must accommodate. These include 'part of' relationships, optionality and iteration. The lettered examples below refer to figure 4.

Most protocols consist of an aggregation of would-be actions, and are said to be *composite,* e.g. F and H. A protocol which is not composite is said to be *atomic,* e.g. G, J, M & I_2. Components of composites are considered protocols in their own right, and are known as *component protocol*s, e.g. G & I_1. A component may itself be composite, e.g. H. The composite protocol directly 'owning' a component is termed its *parent protocol,* e.g. F & H. A parentless protocol - atomic or composite - is known as a *main protocol,* e.g. F, and this is what the would-be protocol user first sees. A component is either *mandatory,* i.e. always implemented if the parent composite is implemented, e.g. G & H, or *conditional,* i.e. only implemented if certain conditions are true, e.g. L, M & N. A protocol may have a component, such as I_2 whose completion is not related in any way to the completion of its direct and indirect parents.

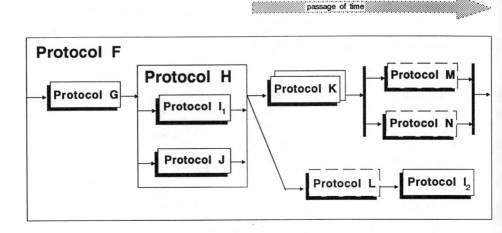

Fig 4 The anatomy of a protocol

The same action type, e.g. 'take a blood pressure', may occur more than once within a composite protocol, but each instance is uniquely identified as a specific component: I_1 and I_2 are such components. A protocol may not recurse, i.e. be a component of itself. A protocol may represent the iteration of a task a fixed or variable number of times, and implementation of such a protocol will produce a number of uniquely identified actions. A protocol, e.g. for a drug treatment, may of course appear - with different identifiers - as a component of any number of main protocols, as well as being a main protocol in its own right.

4.2 Version control

In addition to a unique title, each protocol has at least one *version*, and each version has a *status* - 'under development', 'under test', available', 'superseded' or 'withdrawn'. It is a *version* of a protocol which is actually implemented, and successive versions are said to *supersede* one another. A version of one protocol may be superseded by a version of another protocol, provided that the successor includes the foci and intention of the superseded version. Revision of a protocol implies the production of a new version of the protocol itself, and commonly of all other protocols that include it as a component. In figure 4, the revision of protocol J would result in new versions of H and F. Versions do not preclude the concurrent existence of *different* protocols that deal with the same focus.

4.3 Kinds of protocol

The kinds identified by DILEMMA are shown in figure 5. Currently there are two axes for 'kinds': *protocol intention* and *inference mechanism*. The 'kind of intention' constrains the protocol focus and the outcome. For example it is not possible to 'treat' an unknown subject characteristic, or for a diagnostic protocol to have a result that is not of the class 'diagnosis'. The intention kinds include enabling and planning action types directed towards a particular

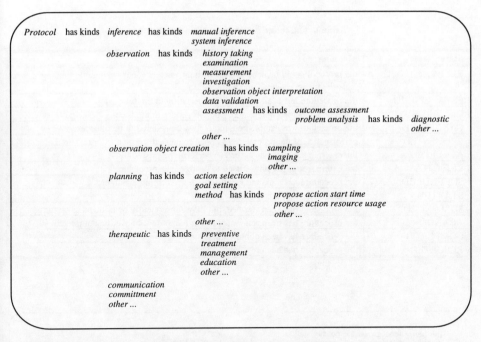

Figure 5 Protocol kinds identified by DILEMMA

subject, as well as actions that are obviously clinical. Protocol kinds equate to the concept type *protocol intention* and also the concept *action type*. Procedures inherit the kinds of the protocol which spawned them.

5 Describing the behaviour of a protocol

Having represented the static elements of a protocol, it is now necessary to describe the dynamic aspects of protocol implementation. Implementation is carried by the *protocol task manager* using the concepts *action state*, *state transition* and *state transition criterion*.

5.1 Action states, (action) state transitions and (action) state transition criteria

At any one time, a procedure generated as a result of implementing a protocol must be in one of the *action states* shown in table 1. All kinds of action - and therefore procedure - cannot assume all possible states. For example, the 'relevant' state can only apply to a main procedure or a conditional component, and an inference protocol cannot assume the 'requested', 'accepted' and 'rejected' states. Even where a state is valid for a procedure type, the protocol author may elect not to use it: he or she might only use the 'reported' state for a procedure always established and performed by a clinician within a single consultation.

Only a subset of the transitions between states can sensibly occur, and these are shown in figure 6. The execution of a procedure is controlled and recorded by means of *state transitions*, and the two mechanisms provided in the DGPM to achieve this are the *state transition criterion* and *user authorisation*. Each transition destination state has one state transition criterion, which represents a statement which must be true before that transition can be proposed. Most proposed state transitions will require explicit authorisation from one or more agents (in some cases including the patient or a proxy) before they may

Table 1 The complete set of possible action states

State	Meaning
RELEVANT	the protocol could be used to deal with the current focus & intention being considered, and has become a procedure
ESTABLISHED	the procedure has been chosen for application to the focus
DISCARDED	it has been decided not to apply the procedure to the focus
CANCELLED	the procedure was established, but is now considered to be unnecessary
REQUESTED	performance of the procedure has been requested from an external supplier
ACCEPTED	the external supplier has agreed to perform the procedure
REJECTED	the external supplier has refused to perform the procedure
SCHEDULED	the procedure has a planned start time, a performing agent, etc.
STARTED	the procedure has been started
SUSPENDED	the procedure has been stopped, but may subsequently be allowed to continue
ABANDONED	the procedure has been scheduled or started, but will never be completed.
COMPLETED	the procedure has been completed
REPORTED	the procedure has been reported

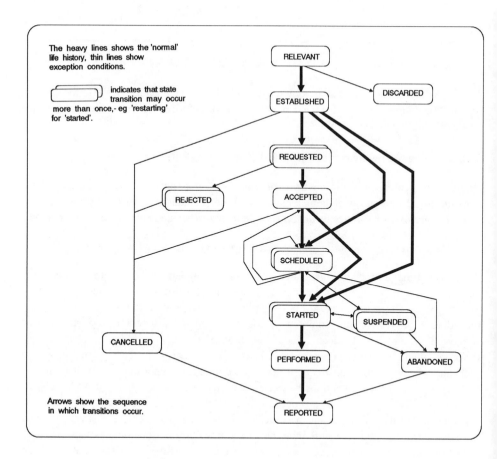

Figure 6 Possible action (and procedure) life cycles

proceed, and will be offered for authorisation (or refusal) by the user(s). The user may always change the state of a procedure explicitly via the protocol manager, but only as permitted by the protocol definition. Each criterion may involve a conjunction or disjunction of conditions and sub conditions, comprising patient characteristics and state transitions of other protocols, optionally with temporal qualification.

5.2 Choosing a main protocol to implement

The birth of a procedure takes place in two steps. Firstly the protocol's *relevance criterion* is used to assess the relevance of each protocol to the focus presented to it, building a list of any suitable candidates. Secondly - if the list is not empty - possible arguments are derived about the suitability of each relevant protocol from its *establishment criterion*, by checking the patient record for the presence of the facts that favour or disfavour its use, and using the results of that process plus *protocol outcome* data to inform user choice. Often the protocol task manager will not propose that choice, as it involves values (e.g. patient preferences) outside the application system, and/or parameters which are incommensurate. In such cases the role of the protocol manager will be restricted to supplying the application with the data relevant to making that choice. The outcome of protocol selection will be either one protocol which is to be applied to the patient and the discarding of any other relevant ones, or the discarding of all relevant protocols.

5.3 The protocol relevance criterion

Each relevance criterion must have one or more *inclusion parameter*, and zero or more *exclusion parameters*.

The *inclusion parameters* must include identify at least one *focus* - 'indication for use' in clinical terms - for which the protocol offers some form of benefit. Each focus will have one *intention* associated with it, e.g. 'to treat', 'prevent', 'manage', 'observe', 'diagnose', etc. The intention is constrained by the focus type: thus a focus consisting of a patient characteristic classed as 'unknown' would always be associated with an intention 'to observe' it. Taken together, problem and intention define the goal or purpose of the protocol, i.e. 'to treat stage II breast cancer'. The eligibility criterion will also identify any *necessary features* which the subject - e.g. patient - must possess to qualify as a suitable candidate for application of the protocol, or that the organisation performing the protocol will need.

The *exclusion parameters* - contraindications in clinical terms - record features which preclude the use of a protocol in both main and component roles. For example, breast cancer treatment protocols including teratogenic chemotherapy would be contraindicated by concurrent 1st trimester pregnancy, and some would be contraindicated for treatment of (the rare) cases of breast cancer in men. Some contraindications, e.g. 'having diabetes mellitus' last for life, whilst others - notably those due to an ongoing intervention, such as the administration of a drug - may be stopped or changed so that the protocol is no longer contraindicated. Only 'permanent' exclusion parameters will therefore result in the protocol being considered irrelevant: the user will be allowed to explicitly override non-permanent exclusions during protocol selection and afterwards, but not at the start transition or - if there is not one - at the transition preceding starting.

5.4 An example of a protocol relevance criterion in declarative form

The following shows a declarative representation of a relevance criterion. The first part contains the knowledge needed for main protocol FB01 to become 'relevant'. The second part is the generic rule that uses this knowledge. It can readily be represented by a symbolic decision procedure, and has been implemented in the DILEMMA protocol task manager. The link "*suggests_relevance_of*" links problems - e.g. indications of use or foci - to actions that are relevant to the problem. 'Intention' is not used in the rule, but could easily be so if required.

```
fact("has eligibility criterion","FB01","FB01 eligibility criterion").
fact("define","FB01 eligibility criterion","FB01 eligibility set").
fact("member","FB01 eligibility set","FB01 problem").
fact("member","FB01 eligibility set","FB01 intention").
fact("member","FB01 eligibility set","FB01 necessary feature criterion").
fact("member","FB01 eligibility set","FB01 exclusion criterion").
fact("define","FB01 problem","FB01 problem set","min",1).
fact("define","FB01 necessary feature criterion","FB01 necessary feature set","min", 2).
fact("define","FB01 exclusion criterion","FB01 exclusion set","max",0).
fact("member","FB01 problem set","stage 1 breast cancer").
fact("member","FB01 problem set","stage II breast cancer diagnosed in last month").
fact("define","FB01 intention","to treat").
fact("member","FB01 necessary feature set","age > 30").
fact("member","FB01 necessary feature set","sex female").
fact("member","FB01 exclusion set","pregnancy").
fact("member","FB01 exclusion set","body-mass index low").
fact("member","FB01 exclusion set","poor general condition").
```

```
If "current patient" has_patient_record "current problem"="problem"
    and "problem" has_type "problem class"
    and "problem class" suggests_relevance_of "clinical task"
    and "clinical task" has_proposal_link "protocol proposal link"
    and "protocol proposal link" exists_between "problem" and "protocol"
    and "eligibility criterion" of "protocol" has_truth_status "TRUE"
then "protocol" makes_transition_ to_state "relevant"
```

5.5 Selecting the 'best' relevant protocol

Although the selection criterion will be 'null' where selection is to be done manually, there will usually be one or more *selection parameter* that provides data relevant to the selection decision. A selection parameter may be a subject characteristic, an action state or a resource, with or without temporal qualification, and can play one of a number of roles.

Exclusion parameters act as they do in a relevance criterion, the user having the option to explicitly ignore them as described above in section 5.3.

Where a protocol is of the therapeutic kind, *protocol outcome parameters* allow the user to assess the benefit the protocol offers vis-à-vis the 'do nothing' option represented by the focus prognosis. This may be based on information specific to the subject, but commonly the only data available will be about populations, i.e. those with the focus problem or those who have been treated with the protocol in the past.

Pro and *con parameters* represent facts which if present favour or disfavour the use of the protocol, but which do not mandate or preclude its use. Typical cons for an drug administration protocol would be the 'cautions' given in many formularies, whilst a patient record item indicating successful use of the drug for previous treatment of the focus problem would be a pro parameter.

Ranking parameters cover facts which can only be assessed in relation to those of any other relevant protocols, such as the 'average cost of implementation'.

Eligibility and selection parameters must be consistent within themselves and with each other. For example, an indication for use of a protocol may not also be used as a contraindication of that protocol or its components.

5.6 *Controlling movement of an established procedure through the remaining states.*

The remaining states - see figure 7 - can apply to main or component protocols, subject to the common-sense constraints imposed by the type of the procedure described above in section 5.1. The transitions of the remaining states differ only in the parameter types which their transition criteria can use. The types permitted include:

- subject characteristics
- action state transitions
- protocol target parameters
- protocol input resource parameters.

Any of these may be temporally qualified.

A state transition of a composite protocol can either entail, or be entailed by, state transitions of one or more of its components. These entailments can be stated as universal rules, which can be embedded in the protocol task manager. One the most likely uses of composite state transitions is as a shorthand way of getting all components in a relevant state to make the transition to an exception state, i.e. 'cancelled', 'abandoned' and 'suspended'. Transitions to these states require the user to consider supplying the reason for the transition if - as may well be the case - the transition is requested by the clinician rather than proposed by the governing state transition criterion.

5.7 *Controlling the sequence in which component protocols are implemented*

State transition criteria not only allow us to select main protocols and to control procedure life cycles, they also enable us to define the succession relationship between protocol components. A succession relationship between component procedures is expressed by means of a transition criterion for an action which includes the triggering state transition in an earlier action as one of its parameters. In the simplest - and commonest - case, completion of one component allows another component to start. Detection of a triggering event (i.e. a 'preceding' state transition in another protocol or a patient data item mentioned in the criterion) will cause the protocol manager to evaluate the condition of its potential successor(s) in full. The condition may be found to be satisfied immediately, or it may become satisfied at a subsequent time as a result of a subsequent event.

Mention of a specific predecessor in several subsequent components' state transition criteria allows the predecessor to have more than one successor component, and - unless they are all mutually exclusive - allows two or more of these to be performed in parallel. Conversely, execution of a component protocol may be triggered by state transitions of more than one possible predecessor, either as exclusive alternatives or in combination. This will be indicated by including each necessary component state as a part of the state transition criteria for the triggering of a state transition in the successor protocol. Thus a component protocol for discharging an inpatient might only be able to start when all the parallel strands of activity involved in the treatment have attained the 'reported' state.

The implementation (or otherwise) of conditional procedures is governed by their establishment criterion: such activities are typically implemented upon the appearance of a particular subject characteristic. If the conditional activity is one of set of exclusive alternatives for which no establishment transition criterion is supplied, the clinician will be shown the set of alternatives and asked to pick one. Where relevant help may be offered from hypermedia knowledge sources.

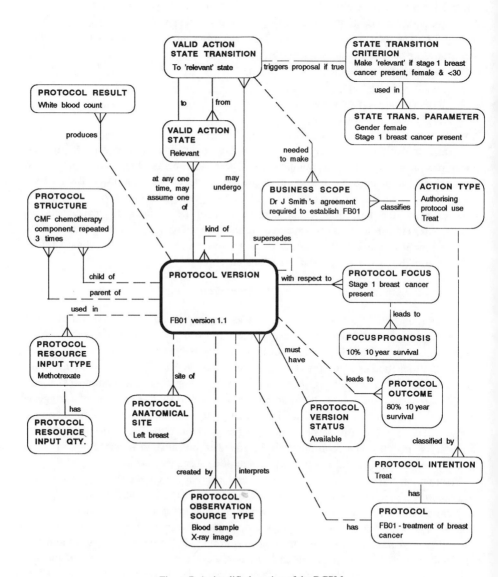

Figure 7 A simplified version of the DGPM

5.8 A look at the overall conceptual model.

Figure 7 shows a 'cut down' version of the Dilemma Generic Protocol Model, using the symbols described in figure 3. For the sake of clarity, much detail about state transition parameters, protocol outcomes and focus prognoses, plus most 'type' concepts, have been omitted. Concepts that have titles not starting with the word 'protocol' (other than 'focus prognosis') are not specific to the DILEMMA protocol model. The resource-related concepts *protocol resource input type* and *protocol resource input quantity* are place holders for further modelling work that is necessary on resource management. The relationship between the agents who can authorise procedure state transitions and the transitions themselves is effected through the concept *business scope,* although the relationship from *business scope* to *agent* has been left out of the diagram to save space.

The concept type *refined version concept* allows a protocol which is used as a component of more than one parent to have 'kinds' of certain concepts used in the original version definition. The most obvious use of this facility would be to allow generalised specification of *protocol resource input*s at version level which are then fleshed out for each use of the version in another composite protocol, but it may also apply to *protocol focus, focus prognosis* and *protocol outcome.*

Some of the relationships shown are restricted to certain types of protocol, but again it is not possible to show the constraints on one small diagram. For instance, only an observation protocol can have a *protocol result,* and only an intervention protocol can have a *protocol outcome* and *focus prognosis.* However in practice this differentiation may be

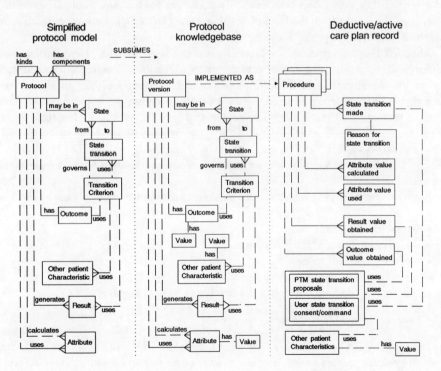

Figure 8 Simplified semantics of the protocol model, protocol knowledge base and patient record

less useful than it seems, as a composite protocol may include actions with different intentions, not all of which the author chooses to explicitly represent as components.

Figure 8 summarises the relationship between the DGPM, a knowledgebase containing specific protocols and the record of the implemented protocol in the patient record. The concepts and inter-concept relationships used in each specific protocol must be an instance of the concepts and relationships contained in the DGPM. The relationship of a specific protocol to the patient record is complicated by the fact that a protocol may well be incompletely implemented, components being discarded, modified or replaced, and extra actions performed. The diagram does not attempt to represent the local tailoring which is almost certain to be applied to protocols developed elsewhere before they are put into use, or the associated development of the local knowledge required about who may authorise the various state transitions involved.

6 Summing up

6.1 Limitations of protocol-based decision support

A protocol is a deterministic process concerned with answering the question 'what should I do?' It is as sound as the knowledge of its authors, and its granularity is determined by the knowledge that its authors can expect the user of the protocol to possess, and the behaviour which the authors wish to encourage. A surgeon describing a process for his peers would take as read things that he would explicitly document for his junior colleagues. On the other hand, he would go to the level of detail necessary to explicitly represent those actions which he wished to see performed more uniformly.

Although they may include conditional elements, it is doubtful if *any* protocol *ever* caters for all the events that could occur during its execution. Concurrent implementation for an individual patient of multiple protocols and interventions that are not protocol-related, plus the presence of unrelated co-morbidity, require the application of general medical reasoning to resolve any interactions that may be generated. For these reasons alone, we see *protocols as providing decision support, not decisions: clinicians - and in some cases patients as well - are ultimately responsible for providing what care is provided, and so for accepting or rejecting most decisions proposed by a decision support system.*

But with that proviso in mind, and for the foreseeable future, protocols are a sound way of:

- disseminating expertise
- providing relevant, consistent, high-quality care
- getting value for money
- auditing past care
- generating data from which to develop future, better clinical practice.

6.2 'A managed process of convergence'

As the paper by Ian Purves in this book shows, there is a small but significant and growing body of evidence that the use of telematics can improve protocol authoring, take-up and the effectiveness of their implementation, despite the known inadequacies of current software.

There is therefore a need to provide telematic tools to assist protocol authors, distributors, implementors, and those investigating the results of their use.

A prerequisite for progress in these areas is an ontology for protocols that enables them to be reused, and that can support links with the other telematically-provided knowledge bases that are needed and that are slowly becoming available, such as drug formularies, diagnostic aids and specialist medical hypermedia products. Protocols will also make new demands of the electronic record, as figure 8 demonstrates.

Several other AIM projects are heavily involved with protocols, and DILEMMA are currently discussing the protocol model with the GALEN and NUCLEUS projects with a view to devising a consensus version of the DGPM and providing better representations of it. The DILEMMA work already shows a strong convergence with that of RICHE approach, largely as a result of a common CBS content. These are first steps in a timely process that should:

- result in an essential element of the telematics infrastructure for the 4th Framework
- pave the way for a pre-standard proposal for submission to CEN TC 251
- generate a protocol ontology that is compatible with that of general medical knowledge
- ensure that the evolving electronic patient record structure can support protocol use.

Acknowledgement

This paper is published by kind permission of the DILEMMA consortium. The organisations involved are:

Advanced Computation Laboratory, Imperial Cancer Research Fund, London, UK

General Practice Research Group, Imperial cancer Research Fund, Oxford, UK

Hewlett-Packard Research Laboratories, Bristol, UK

Royal Brompton National Heart & Lung Hospitals, London, UK

Fondation Bergonié, Bordeaux, France

The NHS Information Management Centre, Birmingham, UK

Deutsches Krebsforschungszentrum, Heidelberg, Germany

MDA Group, Linköping University, Sweden

UNINOVA, Lisbon, Portugal

WOK (CQAR), Nijmegen University, Netherlands

References

[1] The DILEMMA Generic Protocol Model, version 2.1. The DILEMMA Project, London October 1994

[2] The DILEMMA Generic Protocol Model version 2.1 Glossary. The.DILEMMA Project, London, October 1994

[3] The DILEMMA Generic protocol Model Problems and Requirements List. The DILEMMA Project, London, October 1994

[4] J Huang, J Fox, C Gordon, A Jackson-Smale. Symbolic Decision Support in Medical Care. *Artificial Intelligence in Medicine*,5(5) 1993, 415-430

[5] The CBS in 1994. NHS Information Management Centre. Birmingham, UK, 1992.

[6] Gordon C, Herbert S, Jackson-Smale A. Care Protocols and Healthcare Informatics. *Technology and Informatics* (**10**) *Artificial Intelligence in Medicine,* IOS Press, 1993, 289-309

[7] Herbert S, Gordon C, Jackson-Smale A, Renaud-Salis J-L. Protocols for Clinical Care. *Proceedings of 12th International Congress of the European Federation for medical Informatics*, Lisbon, Portugal, 1994 30-35

[8] J Fox, C Gordon, A J Glowinski and M O'Neil, Logic engineering for knowledge engineering: The Oxford System of Medicine, *Artificial Intelligence in Medicine* **2** (1990), 323-339.

[9] Tu S W, Kahn M G, Musen M A, Ferguson J C, Shortliffe E H, Fagan L M. Episodic Skeletal-Plan Refinement Based on Temporal Data, *Communications of the ACM* 32(12) (1989), 1439-1455.

[10] Shortliffe E H, Scott A C, Bischoff M B, Campbell A B, Van Melle W, Jacobs C D, Oncocin: An expert system for oncology protocol management. *Proceedings of IJJCAI*, 81, Vol 1, 876-881 (1981).

[11] The Common Basic Specification Generic Model, version 2.0, 3 vols. NHS Information Management Centre. Birmingham, UK, 1992.

[12] The clinical view of the Common Basic Specification: the COSMOS project clinical process model version 2.0. NHS Information Management Centre. Birmingham, UK, 1993.

Primary Care

Computerized Guidelines for Preventative Care in General Practice

Wilfried Boon[a], Roberto Nardi[b], Stephano Bertelli[c]

[a] Landelijke Huisartsen Vereniging, P.O. Box 20056, 3502 LB Utrecht, The Netherlands
[b] Società Italiana di Medicina Generale, corr.: Via Porta 52, 21050 Bisuschio, Italy
[c] PRISMA Informatica SA, Piazza di Bellosguardo 11, 50124 Florence, Italy

Abstract. Computer-based guidelines for preventative care is an example of the way in which protocols can be put to use in an effective and useful way. However, computerised medical protocols will only be used on a large scale if they are integrated with the computer-based medical record.

The AIM-project ISAAC is working on the development of integrated tools for use in Primary Health Care, and especially General Practice. One of the tools under development is prevention.

In this article, prevention is used as an example of the implementation of protocols. After a short definition of prevention, the implementation of preventative modules (or protocols) in the ISAAC GP information system is discussed.

There are several conditions or critical factors if the implementation of prevention (and protocols) in a GP information system and in a GP practice is to be successful.

In the discussion, some of the opportunities that are emerging with the use of information systems and telematics in primary health care are also discussed, together with the potential of ISAAC and the crucial role that must be played by healthcare providers.

1 Introduction

The target-area of the AIM-project ISAAC (Integrated System Architecture for Advanced primary Care) is Primary Health Care (PHC). The focus of ISAAC is General Practice.

The care that is provided in General Practice is continuous and comprehensive. A GP must deal with acute problems, but is also providing care for the chronically ill. A GP is the care provider with the most knowledge of a patient's background: medical history, family history, work and socio-economical environment. The GP has an advising and coordinating role in the care provision by other health care professionals. The GP is the guide for patients throughout the healthcare system, and in many countries, the GP acts as the gatekeeper in health care.

The tasks of the GP are changing. There is the tendency to promote shared care between the GP and a specialist in the treatment of patients, especially for the chronically ill. Prevention is seen as a very important task of the GP, as is quality assurance. In The Netherlands, the development of GP standards by the Dutch College of General Practitioners supports the changing responsibilities of GPs.

1.1 ISAAC

Important workpackages of ISAAC are the Functional Reference Model, the Integration Architecture, the workpackage dealing with prevention and research, and the workpackage on education and training of both the GP and patients.

Functional Reference Model. The Functional Reference Model (FRM) describes what General Practice in Europe is, through a survey that has been held in 19 European countries. The FRM describes the differences and similarities of General Practice.

To allow the link with information technology, the FRM contains the ISAAC accreditation list. The accreditation list is a detailed list of functional requirements, that can act as a check-list for GP information systems developers and users.

Integration Architecture. The Integration Architecture is a set of (technical) tools that allow a functionally integrated exchange of information. It is dealing with the technically different ways of data transfer between different types of hosts, and provides translation functions which will enable a seamless import and export of medical data into and out of the computer-based patient record.

The Computer-Based Patient Record (CBPR). The core of ISAAC is the CBPR. Much effort has been put in the definition of a well-structured patient record. This is essential if the information contained in the record is to be used for other purposes than "direct care". E.g. coupling with supportive tools requires a stand-alone analysis of patient-data, which is quite different from a GP interpreting data. The patient record must be sufficiently structured to recall not only when, but also why things happened. Relations between the different data-items must be made explicit. Finally, for unambiguous interpretation, the information contained in the CBPR must be linked to standardised terminology.

Only if these conditions for a good CBPR are met, will the record provide the basis for support of the GP.

1.2 Purpose of protocols

There are different purposes for which protocols can be used:

Standardised care. Protocols are an aid for achieving standardised care. A protocol may describe necessary steps, necessary activities and the time-frame in which these activities should be performed.

Quality of care. Protocols can be a major instrument to enhance the quality of care. Protocols provide a way to implement state-of-the-art care into general practice. State-of-the-art, not in the sense of technically advanced, but reflecting the most recent scientifical knowledge on specific subjects.

Protocols may serve as guidelines, e.g. for good clinical practice. In this sense they are helpful in the quality assurance process. And vice-versa, quality assessment can be performed by analyzing the GP's adherence to the standard.

Shared care. Protocols will support the GP in the care of the chronically ill, and in doing so help to move care from specialized care in hospitals to general practice.

In this paper, protocols for preventative care in General Practice are used to illustrate the subject. After an introduction about prevention itself, the potential of computer support in preventative care provision by GPs is described. As examples, Diabetes Mellitus and Influenza Vaccination are presented, as well as a general protocol for screening.

2 Prevention

In the ISAAC project, one of the workpackages is devoted to the implementation of preventative care in General Practice. Prevention is often divided into three levels: primary, secondary and tertiary prevention. However, the borders between the different kinds of prevention are not so clear-cut. From a GP's point of view they may be considered as a continuous process.

2.1 Primary prevention

Primary prevention aims at preventing the disease process from starting. Primary prevention is dealing with the elimination of the factors that are known to play a role in development of a disease. These factors may be very diverse: social status (housing, income, education, employment), lifestyle (smoking, drinking, etc.), "agents", but also predisposing factors or biological events.

The activities of the GP in primary prevention are based on risk assessment. Examples are patient counselling and immunization.

Patient counselling. There are several diseases which have risk-factors that are related to life-style, such as smoking, drinking, diet etc. The aim of patient counselling is to inform patients at risk about the consequences of e.g. their specific lifestyle. They can thus be persuaded to change their behaviour.

A GP will not have time to discuss these factors with all patients. Recognition of specific risk-factors will help to address only those patients who need it. This opportunistic screening can be done during a patient encounter, or in preparation of patient encounters.

Immunization. Immunization is an important part of the healthcare that is provided to (small) children. It is generally done at specific ages. Immunization is often performed by community health services, rather than by GPs.

Other types of immunization are event-triggered, e.g. in the case of tetanus, or in case of travel to areas where specific diseases are endemic. There may be protocols available for these types of immunization.

In some cases, immunization is advised for patients with specific characteristics, e.g. age or disease profiles, as is the case for influenza vaccination. The risk-profile of a patient population is assessed, resulting in a specific patient sub-population that can be addressed for a specific purpose. Those patients who are eligible for vaccination can then be requested to attend specifically appointed consultations where they may receive a vaccination. The use of a computer system makes this follow-up easy, via direct mailing.

2.2 *Secondary prevention*

Secondary prevention aims at the early detection of diseases. Early diagnostics may lead to early treatment, preventing a disease from becoming symptomatic, or avoiding or delaying the occurrence of complications. The benefit for the patient will be a more stable quality of life, and - probably - less severe therapy. The prevention of complications, and limiting the severity of the disease will also result in overall less costly treatment.

Screening a population for risk factors or early symptoms will be the way in which secondary prevention will be carried out. For those patients at risk, specific diagnostic procedures can be carried out, e.g. measuring the blood glucose levels in patients with an elevated risk for Diabetes Mellitus.

2.3 *Tertiary therapy*

Tertiary prevention is performed when a disease has been diagnosed, in order to slow down or avoid its further progress or the development of any possible serious complication. Protocols are of help here, as they will prompt the GP to the proper actions, at the proper time. Tertiary prevention also focuses on the stimulation of patient compliance.

3 Implementation

This section contains a description of the way in which support for the different prevention levels can be implemented [1].

3.1 *Primary prevention*

Risk-assessment can be performed by screening the CBPR for existing risk-factors. This can be done for an individual patient, as well as for the whole practice population. In this example, the risk-factors are shown that define a patient population, eligible for influenza vaccination. The list of ICPC-codes is derived from the Dutch standard on prevention and treatment of influenza [2].

The criteria for Influenza vaccination are: functional disorders of airways and lungs, diseases that may lead to decompensatio cordis, Diabetes Mellitus, chronical renal insufficiency, chronical infection with staphylococcus, and a weakened immune system (HIV, marrow-bone transplants, radiotherapy, and chemotherapy).

With patients over 65, a broader interpretation of the indications is advised.

In ISAAC, the ICPC is used for the classification of diagnoses. In Table 1, the ICPC-codes are listed that can be applied for identification of patients who may be contacted for an influenza vaccination.

3.2 *Secondary prevention*

For the implementation of secondary prevention, two examples are given: the early detection of Diabetes Mellitus, and practice screening.

Diabetes Mellitus

The first example is taken from the Dutch standard on the treatment of Diabetes Mellitus. For Diabetes Mellitus, secondary prevention will be a combination of risk-assessment and proper diagnostic measurements. Table 2 shows a list of risk-factors. These are a combination of diagnoses from the patient's medical history, and measurements.

Table 1: ICPC-codes for the identification of risk-patients with an indication for Influenza-vaccination

ICPC-code	Description	ICPC-code	Description
K74	angina pectoris	R84	malignant neoplasm bronchus/lung
K75	acute myocardial infarction	R85	other malign. neoplasms respir. tract
K76	other / chronic ischaemic heart dis.	R91	chronic bronchitis / bronchiectasis
K77	cardiac failure	R95	emphysema / COPD
K78	atrial fibrillation and flutter	R96	asthma
K79	paroxysmal tachycardia	S10	furuncle / carbuncle / cellulitis local.
K80	ectopic beats	T90	Diabetes Mellitus
K82	cor pulmonale [chronic]	U88	glomerulonephritis, nephr. syndrome
K83	non-rheumatic valve disorder NOS	U99	other disorders of urinary system
K84	other heart disorders		

Once a patient has been identified to be at risk for Diabetes Mellitus, blood glucose levels must be measured, preferably several times. In Table 3, the diagnostical criteria are shown. The blood glucose levels must be interpreted in the context of the presence or absence of evident complaints [3].

Table 2: Some risk-factors for Diabetes Mellitus

Family history of Diabetes Mellitus
Body Mass Index >30
Hypertension
Cerebrovascular diseases
Hyperlipidaemia

Table 3: Diagnostic criteria for Diabetes Mellitus

Measurements		
Measurement	Normal	Abnormal
blood glucose fasting	5.5 mmol/ml	6.7 mmol/ml
blood glucose 2 hrs	7.7 mmol/ml	11.2 mmol/ml
Interpretation		
1. Diabetes Mellitus when no complaints are present, and 2 abnormal glucose values have been found.		
2. Diabetes Mellitus when there are evident complaints, and 1 abnormal glucose value has been found		

Table 4 General screening activities for the whole population

Subject												
alcohol	15	20	25	afterwards if necessary								
smoking	15	20	25	afterwards if necessary								
drug abuse	15	20	25	afterwards if necessary								
sex. behaviour	15	20	25	afterwards if necessary								
blood pressure	15	20	25	30	35	40	45	50	55	60	annual	
breast exam	15	20	25	30	35	every 2 yrs		50	annual			
weight/diet	15	20	25	30	35	40	45	50	55	60	65	70
testis exam	15	afterwards as suited to assessed risk										
pap test	start sex. act.			30	every 2 yrs			50	annual			
gyneacol.	menarche			30	every 2 yrs			50	annual			
breast exam						40		50	every 2 yrs			
ecg				30		40		50		60	65	70
oto-rhino-laryngal	15			30		40		50		60	65	70
eye exam	15			30		40		50		60	65	70
urologic exam						40		50	55	60	65	70
lipids	15			30		40		50		60		70
glucose	15			30		40		50	55	60	65	70
uric acids	15			30		40		50		60		70
occult blood	15			30		40		50		60		70
other	15			30		40		50		60		70

Screening of practice population

The second example deals with the screening of a practice population, and is defined by the Italian GP association SIMG [4]. The list of subjects, and the patient age at which the screening activities should take place, are given in Table 4.

3.3 Tertiary prevention

For Diabetes Mellitus, tertiary prevention consists of regular contacts with the patient. At each contact, a specific list of items is asked. The effect of the therapy is monitored, as is the possible onset of complications. Patient compliance is promoted by asking specifically about any problems occurring with therapy and diet.

Table 5: Treatment of Diabetes Mellitus

every 3 months	every 12 months, additionally:
history	**history**
well-being	pruritus
complaints	pain, tingling extremities
weight development	sexual problems
problems with diet	visus problems
problems with medication	anginous complaints
measurements	claudication
blood glucose level	physical activity
weight	smoking
	physical examination
	inspection feet
	a.dorsalis pedis
	blood pressure
	reflex achilles tendon
	measurements
	creatinine
	cholesterol
	protein in urine

In addition to the items shown in the two rows of Table 5, a bi-annual eye-check should be performed by an ophthalmologist.

4 Technical prerequisites

There are several technical conditions that must be fulfilled before computerised support becomes feasible.

4.1 Integration with the CBPR

Computerized protocols should be really integrated with the CBPR. Only then, the data that are already available can be fetched from this record. Reversely, if the data that are entered in the preventative protocols should also be available in the CBPR, they must be fed back into the CBPR. In both cases, unnecessary retyping is avoided.

Another advantage of integration is, that no extra machines are necessary to use the protocol.

Finally, the integration helps to fit the preventative activities into the daily routine.

4.2 High-quality patient data

Protocols will only operate reliably when the data that are used are reliable. All data must be checked at the point of data-entry, for their syntactical and semantical correctness. This implies that the GP should be responsible for data entry. Only then can mistakes be directly fed back to the "generator" of the information.

Of additional importance for sound interpretation is the use of a standard (controlled) vocabulary. Furthermore, the data must be structured in such a way as to make unambiguous interpretation possible. Therefore, the when and why of activities that have taken place must be known. Temporal and causal relationships must be explicitly available in the CBPR. This can be achieved by using the episode-oriented record paradigm, in combination with the problem-oriented record method.

Systems must be designed in such a way that maximal support is given during the recording process.

5 Organisational prerequisites

The organisational requirements are at least as important to implement protocols successfully as the technical requirements.

5.1 Consensus at a national level

Protocols will only be widely used if a consensus exists about their content. An even wider use will be possible if the consensus is not limited to one professional group, but when the different groups (GPs, specialists) agree on them. This opens up ways for better cooperation. The Dutch standards program, carried out by the Dutch College of General Practitioners is a fine example of a standard that has received wide acclaim, from GPs, from the health ministry and from the public. The success can be largely attributed to the direct involvement of GPs in the development [5].

Moreover, the implementation of standards must be flexible. GPs should not be forced to adhere to the standards: the standards are intended as guidelines. GPs should be able to incorporate their own preferences. In many cases, the consensus standard will be minimal standard. They leave space for the interests of the individual care-provider or group of care providers, and to allow adaptation to local circumstances.

5.2 Support of the practice

Protocols will only be used if (parts of) the extra work, which is unavoidable, can be delegated. Protocols will be helpful here as well, as they may contain guidelines for the ancillary staff. When a patient makes a visit to the GP, related to Diabetes Mellitus, the practice nurse may perform some examinations and ask some of the questions. The GP can subsequently elaborate on this information in the contact with the patient, and concentrate on the aspects to which he is most qualified.

Delegation of tasks to well-trained practice staff will be a step in the right direction, but support of practice management is also necessary: planning of specific consultations, and overviews (practice status, progress, etc.).

5.3 Prevention as a basic GP-task

To allow the introduction of preventative activities on a large scale in general practice, they must be recognised as one of the basic tasks of GPs. GP associations have a task in promoting this view, to provide the necessary educational support, and to take care of the necessary incentives in negotiations with regulating bodies.

6 Discussion

6.1 Opportunities for protocols

The implementation of protocols in General Practice in a computerized way, and the rapid introduction of telematics services open up a wealth of opportunities for the years to come.

Computer-based support. Computer-based support is the only way to make (complex) protocols available and useful in General Practice. A necessary condition, as mentioned previously, is a tight integration with a well-structured, and well-kept, computer-based patient record.

Shared care. Another opportunity that comes to mind is the concept of shared care. Nowadays, too often the care for chronic patients is provided by specialists. Good protocols will allow to move at least part of this (expensive) care to primary care. With the proper use of telematics services, both parties will be informed about the status and progress of a patient. When both parties are similarly well informed, and capable of providing high-quality care, this can only stimulate a more close cooperation between primary- and secondary care. The protocols must contain specific agreements on the responsibilities of the partners involved. The moments to switch care from one provider to the other must be well-defined.

Practice audit and quality assessment. The use of computer-based protocols makes it very easy to perform practice audit in very specific areas. In a broader sense, this should be embedded in a quality assessment program. The effect of introduction of planned preventative activities must be assessed, in terms of better patient health status, reduced occurrence of complications, and cheaper treatment.

6.2 Potential of ISAAC

Open system. ISAAC is an open system. The integration architecture takes care of this. This means that integration with protocols can be achieved easily, and that exchange of information with other care providers (shared care!) is technically possible. The organisational barriers, however, may prove to be harder to overcome. Finally, ISAAC makes use of existing standards as far as they are available.

Configurability. A part of the ISAAC design strategy is the configuration tool. This makes it easy to make adaptations with respect to the demands of individual users (their preferred ways of working and/or their specific tasks), and in accordance with different national requirements.

There are many differences between the different European countries. This is also true for the protocols that are used for prevention: see for example the Dutch and Italian examples of implementation of secondary prevention in paragraph 3.2. Any protocol system or software must be able to cope with these differences.

Good patient record. The CBPR of ISAAC is based on the episode-oriented approach and the problem-oriented method. Causal relationships are easily made. Standards are used when available.

7 Professional responsibilities

Development of standards. The development of standard guidelines, for prevention, treatment, diagnostic purposes or shared care, must be done by the profession. This will ensure maximum commitment of care providers to the standards. Also, the development of standard vocabularies, standards for data interchange, etc. must also be done by health care professionals. The different sectors in health care (e.g. primary and secondary care providers) must cooperate closely. This will facilitate the shared care concept, and the continuity of care in general.

Implementation. The professional bodies are responsible for the implementation of standards in practice. To achieve this, there must be good relations with user groups and system vendors. This will ensure an adequate implementation of the technical prerequisites. Good relationships with government and payers will help to create the facilities that are necessary to change practice organisation. The funds that are necessary to expand the tasks of GPs and the extra staff must be negotiated.

Education. The professional organisations, together with user-groups and vendors, must put much effort in the education of end-user, in order to realise good recording practice by Gps. The GP who is recording all data in the CBPR must do this in a good way. He must be motivated to do so, it must be clear why a structured record is necessary, and what are the intrinsic benefits of this.

Quality policy. The use of protocols must be linked with the quality policy of the profession. This includes quality assessment, which can be done at the practice level, or at a larger scale.

8 Conclusion

Protocols are a real option in primary health care, when they are available in computerized format, integrated with good CBPRs. The protocols that are needed to implement the preventative activities, as presented here, may seem rather straightforward, but they are based on standards from health care providers (so they are well accepted), they can be easily implemented. With the use of protocols in General Practice, a quality tool is introduced which helps the GP to enhance the way in which care is provided. Shared care is facilitated (protocols can be defined by GP and specialists), and protocols will help to communicate the proper information between GPs and specialists.

Many of the current GP applications contain a computer-based patient record that is not sufficiently structured to allow full integration with computer-based protocols. Within the ISAAC project, much effort is put into the development of a highly structured patient record, as the basis for advanced additional functionalities. ISAAC therefore provides an excellent technical platform for further developments, with its CBPR and its integration architecture.

Besides technical requirements, there are the organizational conditions and incentives, for which the professional associations are indispensable.

References

[1] ISAAC Consortium, SIMG (ed). *Prevention and research specifications.* ISA-315-44-01 (1994)

[2] Van Essen GA, Sorgedrager YCG, Salemink GW, Govaert ThME, van den Hoogen JPH, van der Laan JR. *NHG Standaard Influenza en Influenzavaccinatie.* Huisarts Wet. 1993; 36 (10): 342-246. *(in Dutch)*

[3] Meulenberg F, Thomas S, van der Voort H (eds). NHG standards. *5 Examples of guidelines for general practice.* Utrecht, the Netherlands: Dutch College of General Practitioners, 1993.

[4] Società Italiana di Medicine Generale. Proposal.

[5] Thomas S. *Standard setting in the Netherlands: impact of the human factor on guideline development.* Br J Gen Pract 1994; June, 242-243.

Health Telematics for Clinical Guidelines and Protocols
C. Gordon and J.P. Christensen (Eds.)
IOS Press, 1995

Computerised Guidelines In Primary Health Care: Reflections And Implications

Ian Purves

The Sowerby Unit for Primary Care Informatics, The Medical School,
University of Newcastle, Newcastle-on-Tyne NE2 4HH, UK

Abstract. This chapter introduces the role of clinical guidelines in improving the quality of care in Primary Health Care. It goes on to describe the literature with respect to the development, dissemination and implementation of clinical guidelines while attempting to highlight factors liable to impede their use. It concludes with a discussion of the role of informatics in ensuring the difficulties described are avoided.

1 Introduction

Health care has reached an impasse in its development. The variability in the quality of care has been shown to be immense and the quality is generally poor. The challenge has been made to improve the quality of the care delivered [1]. This comes at a time when we are also starting to understand medical decision making [2] and clinical epidemiology has redefined the *"science of the art of medicine"* [3]. Furthermore a structured approach to reducing the paternalistic nature of health delivery and enhancing self care has been described [4]. The time has come to change the way in which we work that encompasses a change in focus towards the patient, increasing team work and utilisation of up to date medical knowledge to manage each patient.

There still lies ahead a fundamental problem with the exploding nature of medical knowledge [5,6]. Computer based knowledge systems would seem to be the solution [7,8], in parallel with a change in clinical method [9]. However, problems do arise, as it is easy to perpetuate or even increase the paradoxical issue of "data overload" combined with "knowledge underload" [10]. Presenting the clinician with pertinent and easy to assimilate knowledge related to the dilemma that is being faced, with respect to a patient, is the goal [11]. Are computerised guidelines part of the solution in resolving these dilemmas? We need to consider their proven role in reminding clinicians about actions to be taken [12,13] and perhaps their role in helping bad collectors and organisers of patient data [5]. What is the balance between differing focuses for computerised guidelines and how do we successfully implement them ?

2. Improving Health Care With Guidelines?

The initial challenge in any guideline setting program is to define the goal of the program [14]. It is, perhaps, obvious that the goal is improving quality of health care [15-17]. However the context in which guidelines are developed is all important [14] as the hidden goal may be cost containment or boosting the credibility of "expert" opinion, etceteras. The first activity in any guideline program is the development of the guideline [16-18]. There are two issues which need considering; the composition of the guideline setting group and the method of developing the guideline [16].

Grimshaw and Russell, in a systematic review of rigorous evaluations of guidelines, reached a conclusion which is outlined in Figure 1 [16,19]. I have also used Woolf [18] in Figure 1 to further amplify the development strategy (this is the list on the left hand side of the box). The figure presents the process of a guideline program, from development through dissemination to implementation. In each of the three boxes, the higher the strategy on the list, the more probable that it is effective. However, each of the strategies is also flagged with ✔ for acceptable strategy and ✗ for unacceptable strategy from the guideline users perspective (my interpretation). It can be seen that the greater the separation from those who would implement the guideline and the greater the comprehensiveness of the development strategy, the less likely that it will be successful. However it can also be seen that when developing guidelines, a more central approach is the most acceptable, despite reducing "ownership". The centralised strategy will produce a more valid guideline because of the availability of greater skills in guideline development, clinical skills and resources [20]. Clearly, there is little need to "re-invent the wheel". Furthermore guidelines produced locally will be very difficult to evaluate at a national level. Having highlighted that the least effective strategy for development was the only acceptable approach, Grimshaw and Russell's review went on to resolve these difficulties by highlighting successful dissemination and implementation strategies. It is with these two strategies that the role of clinical informatics come to the fore.

An important issue of guideline development is the process necessary to create a guideline which will "improve the quality of health care". Woolf [18] has reviewed the differing approaches and has highlighted four separate approaches (Figure 1 - left side top box). Informal consensus development is the historical approach, with the guidelines based on expert opinion. Formal consensus development is again based on expert opinion but in a more structured way. It is clear that these techniques are potentially quite dangerous as they are dependent on the pre-consensus bias of the "experts" and the "guideline development group" process. Furthermore, it is difficult to document the basis for the recommendations

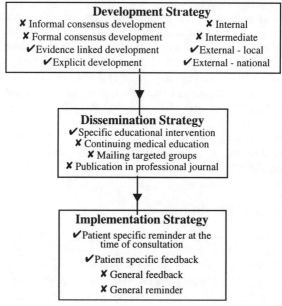

Figure 1: Success vs acceptability of guideline development, dissemination and implementation

and therefore validate them. The two more acceptable approaches to guideline development are evidence based and explicit guideline development. The evidence based approach has been around from 1980 [21]. This approach involves complete literature reviews and attaching the evidence to the guidelines. The main problem with this approach is that much of accepted medical practice has never been validated and therefore strict adherence to this approach leaves gaping holes in the guideline. Eddy [22,23] has more recently presented the explicit approach. In this approach guideline developers specify the benefits, harms and costs of potential interventions and derive explicit estimates of the probability of each outcome. The approach uses evidence and mathematical models in the main but does resort to a documented expert opinion where necessary. The output of this approach is in the form of "balance sheets" [24]. The main difficulty of this approach is that it is complex, very time consuming and therefore expensive. As yet, it has not found its niche in the role of guideline development and the gold standard approach remains the evidence based approach.

To successfully implement centrally developed guidelines, Grimshaw and Russell [19] have indicated that the most successful dissemination strategy was specific educational intervention focused on the content of the guideline and the weight of evidence behind it. This strategy has obvious potential for using informatics techniques in delivering and updating computerised guidelines via telematics and education associated with the process of integrating the guideline into the clinical information system. However, it must be noted that social influence theory tells us that the information contained within a guideline must concur with (or be believed to represent) that of the clinician's peer group [25]. In fact the same is true of guidelines globally; does the peer group value and use them ? The dissemination strategy of specific educational intervention is successful in "Information Transfer" but poor in "Norm Transfer" [25] unless the process involves a group perceived to make up the clinician's peer group or an opinion leader. It is early days in the use of social influence theory and we await publications to help enhance the process of education within dissemination strategies for guidelines. What perhaps is clear, is that the educational process may be different for different groups of clinicians [26]. As with any innovation, rates of uptake will differ across varying groups of individuals [27], with innovators picking things up regardless (only 2.5% of the population); early adopters needing written methods, scientific argument and credible sources; the majority preferring personal sources, opinion leaders, peer activities and reinforcement by social network; and late adopters requiring regulations, laws, incentives or sanctions, practical resources and provisions [26].

With regard to implementing guidelines, patient specific implementation strategies have been found to be the most effective, especially if the patient was present at the time of the intervention. McDonald [12] identified one of the reasons for failure of guidelines as information overload. Patient specific implementation strategies reduce the overload by reminding the clinician about the relevance of the guideline outside of the patient encounter, and, in, a very focused way, just before or within an encounter. The actual delivery of interventions range from paper guidelines within the patients record [28-30], screening of the record for guideline compliance prior to the encounter by trained health care professional [31] and computer [12, 13,32-39], interactive computerised protocols [40-43], graphical presentation of an algorithm on computer [10], critiquing [44-46] and questionnaires (both paper-based and computer-based) [47]. This last paper by Lilford [47] is one of only two studies which compared paper-based with computer-based patient specific implementation of guidelines. The paper found no statistical difference between paper-based and computerised methods. However, I feel that the study had insufficient power to justify its asertion that "*Computerised systems offer no further advantages*". Further, it was clear that like was not compared with like as the computerised protocol was more complex than the paper one [48]. The implications of guideline complexity and potential information overload are likely to make computerization as an integrated component of a clinical information system the most effective means of implementing guidelines [48]. This is born out by the second study looking at paper vs computers [40] which found the compliance with the guidelines to be statistically greater for the computer form. The computer can simplify the use of guidelines by making use of information within the electronic health care record and navigating the algorithm in a "hidden" fashion. This reduces the information that needs assimilating by the clinician and reduces overload.

3 Why Guidelines Can Be Unusable

Guidelines have been around for many years under differing names and guises: Criteria Mapping [49], Algorithms [50], Protocols [51] and more recently Guidelines [52]; yet they are not perceived to be in common use in clinical practice. In fact simple guidelines are in daily use, but more complex guidelines are still rarely used. As mentioned, McDonald [12] feels this is due to information overload and Mittman [25] raised the question of social norms. The issues are obviously complex and in this section an attempt will be made to tease out the problems without focusing on the choice between computerised or paper implementation strategies.

3.1 Clinician Disagreement with the Concept of Guidelines

It has yet to be accepted by the majority of clinicians that guidelines are a "good thing". Many resent the thought of "cookbook medicine" and feel it will reduce the clinician's self respect and could reduce patients' confidence in them [15]. On the same line there are anxieties of becoming unthinking robots [50], "fear of loss of control" [53] and there is "a fear that medical care would become regimented, uninspired, and mediocre if all of the 'art' were removed from medical decision-making" [54]. These are issues about the "social norms" [25]; unfortunately there is little objective evidence as to the prevalence of these feelings. However, in The Netherlands where standard setting is an accepted "social norm", in a randomised sample of 10% (70% response rate) of all general practitioners, 82% strongly agreed that "National standards give a basis for daily work" [55]. There is obviously an important educational issue here for other countries.

3.2 Clinician Disagreement with the Content of Guidelines

Given that a centralised approach to the creation of guidelines is the only practical one [16], there is the issue of "ownership" [17]. This has been discussed at length in the preceding section, as has the issue of "social norms" [25], which needs to be managed if clinicians are to "agree" with the content of guidelines. The issue revolves around specific education which includes peers and opinion leaders. An alarming example of how guidelines disseminated without education are rejected is given by van der Lei [45]. In a study evaluating critiques of hypertension therapy which were based on reviews generated by 9 experts (one of which was the computerised decision support system HyperCritic), 14 randomly selected general practitioners were asked to comment on the critiques. Even where all 9 "experts" were in complete agreement that the critique was highly relevant, only 45% of the GP's agreed that it was relevant. Furthermore, 24% felt that the critique was not relevant or potentially harmful. HyperCritics' critiques were very much in line with the 8 human "experts". This exposes the fact that clinicians are to a degree unaware of, or underestimate the degree of, their lack of knowledge [56].

3.3 Unrecognisable Mismatch between an Algorithmic Process and Clinician Decision Making

Margolis [50] has raised the issue that *"physicians do not think "algorithmically" and therefore can not learn from algorithms"*. He tries to refute this statement by stating that algorithmic thought processes (seemingly hypothetico-deductive reasoning [2,57] in his comments) are an inherent part of medical decision making. However, pattern recognition is the most important part of differentiating problems [58,59]. In this way, algorithms are perhaps ill suited to differential decision making and are more suited to management planning which is much nearer an algorithmic process. Management planning, though, is itself also a subject for pattern-based formulation (ie: "illness scripts" and "instance scripts" [58]).

3.4 Change Management

I have discussed some approaches to change management along with the diffusion of innovation [26,27,60]. Further comments on the problems encountered have been discussed by Shortliffe [53] and Grol [55]. In Grol's paper [55] 44% general practitioners are reported to have felt that *"Routines are too strong to change"*, and as such there were problems implementing the diabetes standard. This problem revolved around the fact that general practitioners currently perform most of diabetic care and much of the standard involved activities which would be devolved to other professionals. However, there would be a financial disadvantage to the general practitioners to consider using nursing staff or using more of their own time. This raises the issue that change management does not only involve the individuals in the system but also the environment in which they work.

3.5 Individual Patient Management Goals Vary for the Same Problem

Guidelines have to be based on the assumption of achieving good outcomes of care. However, as a concept outcomes are population based rather than individual based. The lack of patient centredness could potentially lead guidelines to produce a management plan which would lead to a good "outcome" but would not achieve the "goal" for patient care [15,50,55,61,62]. This is due to the fact that social and psychological components of the patient's problem may justify "under" or "over" management of the problem to achieve the goal for the patients' care (as negotiated between clinician and patient) [63].

3.6 Legal Anxieties About Negligence

Deviations from the guideline to aim for a patients "goal" rather than an "expected outcome" must be legitimate. However, this does cause some anxieties and may lead to legal liability [15,53]. A case for negligence may be possible in court along the lines: "your very own computer advised you to do X and yet you didn't". It is clear the guideline must record the patient's involvement in the decision together with the information based on which the decision was made, if this liability problem is to be avoided.

3.7 Time Constraints within Patient Encounters

On a subjective level I have found that if you try to implement a computerised guideline which is not sensitive to the time constraints of an encounter, it will not be used. Any extra activity involves more time. Furthermore, the time constraints not only vary from day to day, but encounter to encounter (e.g. in the case of the patient who presents with a sore throat but is overdue a review of their ischaemic heart disease - neither the patient or doctor will thank you for a insisting prolonged review at this point). Grol found that 33% of general practitioners had problems with the *"extra time and energy"* needed to use the diabetes standards in his study [55]. Brownridge et al [40] found a 35% increase in the length of encounters when an interactive computerised protocol was used. Clearly guidelines should be sensitive to the available time.

3.8 Local Variations in Management Plans

The environment in which the guideline is to be implemented has been mentioned, together with change management and time constraints. A further angle to this environmental issue is the need for adaptation to local variation in *"constraints and opportunities"* [62,64]. There is obviously a difference between practices which are 2 miles or several hundred miles from a regional speciality centre. There may be lack of equipment (e.g. ECG) or local population demographic issues which entail adjustments to the guideline. These issues need to handled in the dissemination process to ensure the "centralised" guideline can be effectively implemented.

3.9 Ambiguous and/or Illogical Guidelines

To date, there seems to have been little consideration of the implementation strategy during the development of guidelines [17]. Most guidelines are presented in a written form; this has led to ambiguous statements and illogicalities within them. Shiffman has found several examples of this by applying the technique of augmented decision tables [65,66,personal communication], even in guidelines produced by the RAND Corporation [66]. Not only does this technique help with ambiguity and illogicalities but it also reduces the rule set necessary to implement the guideline [65]. However, the role of decision tables should not be overplayed. They are the first area in the literature to highlight need for checking of consistency, feasibility and redundancy. Their role is within a guideline authoring tool which could, for example, also check for data not recorded that is needed and for actions which have no associated rule.

3.10 Consensus Views "Portrayed" as Evidence Based

The issues of consensus vs evidence based guidelines has yet to reach most of those (opinion leaders, innovators and early adopters [26]) who would take notice of this problem. The issue is that *"Guidelines are intellectually suspect: by reflecting expert opinion they may formalise unsound practice"* [15]. For those who do understand the issue, it downgrades the importance of guidelines overall and may be fuel for the "cookbook medicine" argument.

3.11 Data Overload vs Information Underload

Greenes has highlighted that "Physicians today are faced with "data overload" and paradoxically, "information underload" - the inability to locate pertinent, needed knowledge in a sea of data with which they are inundated" [10]. Although guidelines are a very focused form of decision support, they still can be presented in a way which continues to overload the clinician. A paper algorithm with pages of explanation or a guideline published in a journal in a non-clinically sensitive style are a good example of ways to overload the clinician. From a computer perspective guidelines which are presented which are not sensitive to the implementation environment also fall into this trap.

3.12 Potential Rigidity of Current Computer Implementation

There are several forms of implementations of guidelines in the literature (listed above); of these interactive computer algorithms/protocols is one of the most comprehensive of approaches. However, this approach has a potential problem of rigidity of implementation. Two studies [40,42] found that low level, predictable protocols are "boring". The studies also found that clinicians using protocols which were insensitive to the environment (time constraints and the patient as a unique entity) annoying. However even with these attributes the algorithm/protocols improved history taking/data entry. The lesson learned is that as much flexibility as possible should be maintained when implementing a guideline [62]. Furthermore guidelines should concentrate on more complex problem management leaving data entry templates to help with routine problems.

3.13 Challenge of Data Entry

Finally the problem of data entry into the computer during a patient encounter is prominent in many clinicians' minds [53]. This issue needs to be handled by the interface, and minimising the data input is needed. It also raises the issue of pre-encounter patient-computer interaction [9,67] as supplementary approach to the data input needs.

4. Informatics Mission for Guidelines

The chapter so far has presented and discussed the challenges which face anyone trying design a guidelines program. It has become apparent during the discussion of the evidence to date that a computerised approach to guideline implementation is the preferred option. However there are obviously many issues which need to be faced along the way. The rest of this chapter will discuss where the informatics community can help with a clinical guidelines program.

4.1 Informatics Role in Guideline Development

The process of producing guidelines with the selection of the topic, panel members and clarification of the purpose is discussed by Woolf, Grimshaw and Russell, and Grol [16-18]. These three papers go on to describe the activities of collecting the evidence and developing the guideline.

Woolf's [18] "*clarification of purpose*" includes identifying "*the type of providers and practice settings*". This leads to an understanding of the need for modelling the environment in which the guideline is to be implemented. Modelling of the clinical and cognitive processes has been identified in the informatics literature as a vital first step in any decision support program [68-71] and is an important role for the informatics community. As mentioned earlier the guideline implementation needs to be sensitive to time constraints which are imposed by the day's schedule and the clinical process(es) which is (are) the reason for the current encounter. Differing professional groups will have differing sensitivities to these pressures depending how appropriate the guideline's "interruption" to the flow of the encounter is to their role in the patients management plan. It is possible to model these clinical processes for each professional group and use the model to ensure that the guideline is not intrusive. The issue of cognitive modelling [68,71] is, perhaps, as important as the clinical model in ensuring that the guidelines are usable. Having looked at this area, it is my belief that guidelines should avoid differential diagnosis and focus on suggesting and reminding about management actions and assisting with the negotiation (with the patient) of management plans. Guidelines also have the role in ensuring that the necessary data set for delivery of quality care and achievement of goals is recorded in the health record.

The clinical and cognitive models are only part of the overall environmental model as we need to consider the need for local and patient-related variation of the guideline. To enable these sort of adjustments to be made, it is clear we need to know the validity of the evidence behind the rules in the guideline. Several taxonomies [3,72-74] have been created to help with guideline production and implementation (e.g. Table 1 [74]). From our experience in observing research workers extracting citations, using an adapted form of the process described by Sackett [3], we have found these taxonomies are probably inadequate. The whole process of reviewing and grading citations needs modelling to enable a valid, consistent and simplified approach. This activity model should lead directly into a useful taxonomy grading the validity of the evidence. The taxonomy then needs mapping to usable hierarchical parents, of which there are three (Table 2). As can be seen from the table, thepractical purpose of this grading is not only to help the guideline development process but also in the dissemination strategy. The grading can ensure that adjustment of rules is appropriate and that rules with strong evidence behind them are not adjusted. Furthermore,

Table 1: Evidence grading taxonomy [74]

Grade	Type of evidence - description
Ia	Evidence obtained from meta-analysis of randomised controlled trials.
Ib	Evidence obtained from at least one randomised controlled trial.
IIa	Evidence obtained from at least one well-designed controlled study without randomisation.
IIb	Evidence obtained from at least one other type of well-designed quasi-experimental study.
III	Evidence obtained from well-designed non-experimental descriptive studies, such as comparative studies, correlation studies and case studies.
IV	Evidence obtained from expert committee reports or opinions and/or clinical experiences of respected authorities.

Table 2: Hierarchical parents in evidence grading taxonomy

Grade	AHCPR Description [74]	Practical use of grade in dissemination
A	Required at least one randomised controlled trial as part of the body of literature of overall good quality and consistency addressing the specific recommendation.	Do not remove or alter this rule within the guideline as the evidence behind it is very strong (citation(s) and explanation included).
B	Required availability of well-conducted clinical studies but no randomised clinical trails on the topic of the recommendation.	Do not remove or alter this rule within the guideline unless you are an expert in this domain. There is reasonable supportive evidence behind it (citation(s) and explanation included).
C	Indicated absence of directly applicable clinical studies of good quality.	There no good evidence to support this rule and the options presented are a consensus views of the guideline production panel. You may choose what ever you feel comfortable with.

specific education material should accompany these rules to educate the implementors why they should not be adjusted.

Modelling local constraints and opportunities is an important area to consider in centrally produced guidelines as the development team needs to be explicit about what is a legitimate variation. The US Institute of Medicine has highlighted four reasons why local adaptation occurs [62]:

1. Weakness in the guideline or inappropriate for local use;
2. Specific local or organisational objectives or constraints;
3. Strategic judgements to secure practitioner acceptance; and
4. Protection of habit or self interest.

This work needs enhancing and guideline programs need to be sensitive to these potential variations.

The guideline development process has several areas in which informatics can assist the development team. There is the large issue of identifying the evidence pertinent to the guideline being produced. We have found this a problematic area due to the variability in MESH coding [75]. It is extremely difficult to rely on output from focused MEDLINE queries and impossible to manage unfocused queries. The process of focusing a query has been assisted with UMLS [76] but is still dependent on the underlying MESH coding. Work with the US National Library of Medicine is vital if this is to be resolved. Furthermore, there is a role for the informatics community in ensuring that an international clinical trials (published and current) database is created. Further discussion on this area, although interesting, is outside the remit of the chapter.

Informatics support for the development team becomes more interactive with the group once the first drafts of the guideline appear. The guideline needs checking for sensitivity to the clinical process model, at which the guideline is targeted, and it also needs checking for areas where local adjustment may be an issue. The guideline then needs breaking down into rules, then checking for ambiguity and illogicalities. It should also be checked for interactions between actions and action side effects; this may lead to the insertion of extra actions to resolve these problems. Once this first pass has been finished and the guideline development team has reviewed the output, the task of linking the rule to the evidence grade, the evidence and the acceptable variations in the actions can start. These action variations may be driven by potential local variations, weak evidence for the action(s) related to the rule, and/or differing patient preferences. The patient preferences are much the more complicated issue [77] and can lead to a balance between the evidence and patient preferences which can cause ethical problems for the guideline developers [78]. Although guidelines can not hope to be comprehensive in the coverage of patient preferences it should still be possible to "cover" the majority of possible preferences and goals for patients which are acceptable to the guideline setting group (this of course includes patients). The "coverage" for patient preferences will probably not be within the rules/algorithms of the guideline but in accompanying linked hypermedia. It is important that the educational material used during shared decision making is referenced in the patient's record and that a care pathway with critiquable goal(s) is also entered within the record. It is unlikely that whole process of the shared decision making can be captured other than by what has been described, perhaps supplemented by free text.

At this stage of development the guideline now consists of individual rules which are qualified by the evidence grade, the evidence and potential variations in the appropriate action. It is at this point that the rules need building into clinical process sensitive rule sets. The forms of implementation of these rule sets will be discussed later. Once the first draft of these rule sets has been created, the next task is to prototype the guideline.

The form of prototyping required in this situation is the so called "experimental" type [79]. In this situation the adequacy of the computer implementation is tested by members of the guideline development group and potential users. The prototyping should check how true the implementation is to the guideline and how clinically relevant and usable it is in practice [71,80]. At the moment, in the United Kingdom there are two commercial GP systems with the functionality to implement guidelines; thse use differing user interfaces and knowledge representations. In the absence of a common standard, therefore, prototyping will need to take place on both commercial systems. Clearly any increase of use in computerised guidelines will need a standard knowledge representation, preferably a specification for the interface and any reasoning based on the knowledge (other than algorithm flow). Martin [81] describes the various methods of prototyping and it would seem likely that a step-by-step approach with three interations would be the best approach.

Standards as described will also help with the evaluation of the computerised guidelines. Guideline development should not be a static process [17,18,62]: research produces new information at an ever expanding rate and evaluation of the guideline may identify that it is not achieving its goals. From the current literature it is reasonable to assume that future computerised guidelines will be valid [12,13,33-35,37-40,43, 47,82,83]. However further rigorous trials need to be performed to ensure the proposed techniques are as valid as anticipated. Long term evaluation of distributed guidelines is more pragmatically based on observational data [84-87], although the continued need for rigorous trials has been forcefully put forward [88]. It is important that this debate of rigorous trials vs observational assessment is brought out into the general professional arena, not exclusively the informatics community, and debated at length. Whichever evaluation type becomes the standard, we need to determine the need for access to the data sets which the guidelines record during usage, and which should provide evaluation data. In the United Kingdom we now have a national standard for distributed database queries for general practice, the MIQUEST product [89,90]. This product could easily have its query language (HQL [91]) adjusted to assist in the evaluation process and to be the basis for the collection process for continuous evaluation of computerised guidelines.

This whole guideline development program is a complex process. Yet these programs are becoming ubiquitous. How are we to educate future programs on the relevant research findings and gold standard processes? One technique is Computer Aided Learning (CAL) [92,93]; the advantages of this approach are: a) The use of variety of instructional strategies [94]; b) Use of varied events of instruction c) Learner can be an active participant d) Consistence of instruction e) Time and cost efficiency f) Learner privacy g) Performing task while learning. A CAL package focused on a guideline development program might have the following attributes;

- Creation of program mission (which includes a definition of the indication of use of the guideline);
- Define the objectives and measures of success;
- Selection of guideline setting group;
- Advice on modelling operational environment;
- Search strategy development for acquiring "evidence" to aid domain expert on guideline group;
- Advice on guideline production process;
- Advice on rule set generation from guideline;
- Checking of constancy, feasibility and redundancy;
- Process sensitive rules/algorithms generation with linked hypermedia;
- Advice on rapid prototyping of "interim" guideline;
- Advice on dissemination strategies;
- Advice on evaluation.

4.2 Informatics Role in Guideline Dissemination

At the end of the guideline development program described, the product will consist of clinical process sensitive rule sets and linked hypermedia. The potential for informatics is in the delivery and "personalisation" of these rule sets for the environment in which they will be used. A further role could be in ensuring local "opinion" leaders and the peer group are educated using CAL techniques.

Given the "users" of the guidelines already have a computerised information system, the first phase would be for designated users to "install" the guidelines. This installation process should involve an evaluation of current activity, within the guideline domain, education, personalisation of rules to local needs, and creation of a generic output to install into the users system. To enable assessment of current activity a HQL query [89,90] could be packaged with the computerised rule set to assess current process relating to the guideline domain. The report from this query could be used to identify where variation from the guideline currently occurs. It is likely this would be flagged during a step through look at the rule sets. This step-through activity would also present areas where the rules are based on "weak" evidence and offer options with explanation. It would also identify areas of legitimate local changes to the guideline. In the other "concrete" areas education can be delivered. Having changed the guideline to suit local practice the "installation" can produce a file in "generic" format with which to import into the users system. It can also create a specific educational package based on the rules selected by the installer and those rules which could not be changed. This can then be used internally to inform those not involved with the installation process. The only current example of a generic file format for guidelines is the Arden syntax [95]. This syntax currently falls down because of the lack of a standard medical vocabulary, and each Medical Logic Module (MLM) needs manually editing at each site. There is a potential further problem in that the MLM's bind both knowledge and process together. Although so far I have described clinical process sensitive rule sets, these may not be represented as one module but in two modules with the knowledge and process separated. This separate representation is that chosen by the DILEMMA project [96].

4.3 Informatics Role in Guideline Implementation

The tasks that computerised guidelines perform in aiding the clinician's decisions are as follows:
- Suggesting and reminding about management actions;
- Assisting with the negotiation (with the patient) and recording of management plans and goals;
- Educating the clinician about the evidence behind rule/actions;
- Co-ordinating the team of clinicians along the care pathway (the temporal organisation of interdisciplinary interventions in a patient's management plan) [97-100];
- Ensuring that the necessary data set for delivery of quality care and achievement of goals is recorded in the health record [5].

In order to support the tasks outlined, it is clear that guidelines need implementing in a variety of ways in clinical information systems [10]. The implementation techniques are not exclusive and should be integrated. Furthermore, it is vital they integrate with the patient's computerised health record. Each of these implementation techniques make up the computerised guideline. It is useful to consider computerised guidelines in three dimensions rather than in the usual "flat" view of the algorithm (see Figure 2).

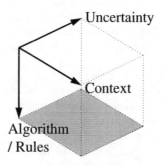

Figure 2: The Three dimensions of computerised guidelines

Each of the dimensions of the computerised guidelines are described further in Table 3. The "up front" dimensions describe the algorithms or rules which can be adjusted according to the context (encounter dynamics; clinical process and patient preferences). Where uncertainty exists, with the clinician or the guideline developers, then this can be resolved by hypermedia links. This third dimension is also a useful metaphor from the interface perspective as users would "drop through" the screen into the hypermedia third dimension to resolve uncertainty.

The process of using a computerised guideline would be as follows:
- Prior to a patient encounter the information system would identify that it had a guideline which matched current patient characteristics (e.g. states or goals). The system would interrogate the electronic record to identify which algorithm or rules were relevant and produce reminders about action(s) or usage of the guideline. Other forms of record critiquing, taken from van der Lei, can be seen in Table 4 [101]. This information is presented on a pre-encounter screen. After a guideline has been used once, the dataset

Table 3: Description of the 3 Dimensions of computerised guidelines

Guideline Dimension	Contents / Description of Guideline Dimension
Algorithm / Rules (*Rule Based/Using Clinical Knowledge*)	• Rules / Algorithms • Care pathway (as a temporal, interdisciplinary map of "standard" care package) • Critiquing model
Context	• Adjustments for the encounter dynamics / clinical process. • Adjustments for patient preferences.
Uncertainty (*Hypermedia Based Clinical Knowledge*)	• Access into explanation of guideline reasoning; to resolve clinician uncertainty. • Guideline development group reached impasse in that there was no evidence to support one action vs another therefore several actions presented with underlying knowledge.

recorded should subsequently assist with the critiquing. If the guideline had not been used then a "screening" [102] form of the guideline could identify the current status of the patient with structured data collection.

→ The critiquing will continue in a dynamic fashion throughout the encounter as data is input. Should the clinician opt to use the guideline interactively(i.e. where this contains more than one ruleor action), the clinician will be queried as the encounter dynamics/clinical process to enable an appropriate rule(s)/algorithm(s) to be selected/adjusted.

→ Once selected, the algorithm will interactively suggest "interim actions" and navigate according to the response, the use of the algorithm will finish with "session end point actions" (see Table 5). During the use of the guideline the clinicians can "drop through" into hypermedia to resolve uncertainty and assist the patient in the process of shared decision making [87]. Further it will leave "navigation lights" within the patients record to enable critiquing and identification of the patients status for the next encounter.

Table 4 - Computer critiquing of the medical record [101]

Type of Task	Content of medical knowledge base	Reports
preparation	rule set of actions which should precede certain clinician's actions	absence of preparation (reminder)
selection	rule set of events which may preclude certain clinician's actions	presence of criteria (alert)
monitoring	rule set of monitoring requirements associated with clinician's actions	absence of monitoring (reminder)
responding	rule set of response-requiring situations associated with clinician's actions	presence of response-requiring situation (alert)

Table 5 - Actions presented in an interactive algorithm

Interim Actions	Session End Point Actions
History taking	Goal setting
Examination	Drug Prescription
Investigation / Procedure	Investigate / observe progression of the problem
	Advise
	Refer
	Procedure
	Plan future encounter

- The guideline will also comprise administration activity which happens independent of an encounter. These critiques will produce patient specific reminders and alerts to ensure that the chosen care pathway is followed.

The computer techniques for implementation have been discussed above; however, it is worth drawing these remarks them together along with the appropriate citations. The simplest form (in the sense of human-computer interaction) of implementation is critiquing using individuals rules [45,46] the types of critique are presented in Table 4; thetable has been created from van der Lei's work [101]. The literature based on one form of critiques, reminders, is the largest for any area of computerised decision support [12,13,32-39]. Grouping the rules into algorithms [10,40-43,102,103] is perhaps the commonest perception of what computerised guidelines are as a concept. The guidelines have great scope as "a framework for decision making and are a starting point for context-sensitive information retrieval" [103]. These algorithms have been presented in a linear text like fashion [41,42] or in a graphical format [10,103]. Abendroth [103] discusses the important issue of the interface; he also highlights the potential for "displaying extremely complex 'algorithms' generated dynamically using an underlying rule base and inference engine" and hints at linkages to further detail outside of the guideline. It is my belief that this "third dimension" or links will consist of hypermedia [104-107] and will enable both clinician and patient education. Using algorithms to guide the completion of "questionnaires"/data sets [47] has also been used, Wyatt [5] highlights the importance of this task. The final technique in implementing guidelines is an overview function which has been presented in Explorer-2 [10]. From the guideline perspective this overview could be centred on the care pathway approach [97,98,100], although as far as I am aware, this has never been implemented.

The final key to implementing computerised guidelines from the informatics perspective is the knowledge representation. If guidelines are to be centrally created and distributed through the dissemination process described we need a telematics standard as a minimum. However if evaluation is not to be supplier specific we also need a standard in knowledge representation and critiquing/inference techniques within all information systems served by the central guideline setting body.

5. Conclusions

This chapter has aimed at pulling together disparate areas of research on guidelines. It has reflected on the issues which research to date has raised, and discussed the implications for the informatics community. It is my belief that guidelines developed, disseminated and implemented in the flexible ways described, will improve the quality of health care. It is now dependent on the three communities of informaticians, guideline developers and social "influence" scientists to pave the way forward.

6. Acknowledgements

I would like to acknowledge the work and support of Martin Eccles, Jeremy Grimshaw, Ian Herbert and Peter Nicklin in helping develop my own thoughts and work on guidelines. I would also like to thank the NHS Management Executive and Northern and Yorkshire Regional Health Authority for funding projects which have led to the views outlined.

References

[1]   Burnum JF. The misinformation era: The fall of the medical record. Ann Intern Med 1989;110:482-484.

[2]   Sox HC, Blatt MA, Higgins MC, Marton KI. Medical Decision Making. Butterworth-Heinemann, Boston. 1988.

[3]   Sackett DL, Hayes RB, Guyatt GH, Tugwell P. Clinical Epidemiology: A Basic Science for Clinical Medicine. 2nd ed. Little, Brown and Company, Boston. 1991.

[4]   Green LW. How physicians can improve patients' participation and maintenance in self-care. West J Med 1987;147(3):346-349.

[5]   Wyatt J. Use and sources of medical knowledge. Lancet 1991;338(8779):1368-1373.

[6]   McWhinney IR. Are we on the brink of a major transformation of clinical method? Can Med Assoc J 1986;135(8):873-878.

[7]   Wyatt J. Computer based knowledge systems. Lancet 1991;338:1431-1436.

[8]   Johnston ME, Langton KB, Haynes RB, Mathieu A. The effects of computer based clinical decision support systems on clinician performance and patients outcome. A critical appraisal of research. Ann Intern Med 1994;120:135-142.

[9]   Purves IN. A computer facilitated clinical method for primary health care. In: Proceedings of North American Primary Care Research Group, Totonto '94. NAPCRG. 1994. (in press)

[10]   Greenes RA. "Desktop Knowledge": A new focus for medical education and decision support. Methods Inf Med 1989;28:332-339.

[11]   Timpka T, Arborelius E. The GP's dilemmas: a study of knowledge need and use during health care consultations. Methods Inf Med 1990;29(1):23-29.

[12]   McDonald CJ. Protocol-based computer reminders, the quality of care and the non-perfectability of man. N Engl J Med 1976;295(24):1351-1355.

[13]   McDonald CJ, Hui SL, Smith DM, Tierney WM, Cohen SJ, Weinberger M, McCabe GP. Reminders to Physicians from an Introspective Computer Medical Record: A Two-Year Randomised Trial. Ann Intern Med 1984;100:130-138.

[14]   Hayward RS, Laupacis A. Initiating, conducting and maintaining guidelines development programs. Can Med Assoc J 1993;148(4):507-512.

[15]   Delamothe T. Wanted: guidelines that doctors will follow. Implementation is the problem. Br Med J 1993;307:218 (Letter).

[16]   Grimshaw J, Russell IT. Achieving health gain through clinical guidelines. I: Developing scientifically valid guidelines. Quality in Health Care 1993;2:243-248.

[17]   Grol R. Development of guidelines for general practice care. Br J Gen Pract 1993;43:146-151.

[18]   Woolf SH. Practice Guidelines, a New Reality in Medicine. Methods of Developing Guidelines. Arch Intern Med 1992;152:946-952.

[19]   Grimshaw JM, Russell IT. Effect of clinical guidelines on medical practice: a systematic review of rigorous evaluations. Lancet 1993;342:1317-1322.

[20]   Brook RII. Practice Guidelines and Practicing Medicine. Are They Compatible? JAMA 1989;262, No. 21:3027-3030.

[21]   White LJ, Ball JR. The clinical efficacy assessment project of the American College of Physicians. Int J Technol Assess Health Care 1985;1:169-174.

[22]   Eddy DM. Clinical decision making: from theory to practice. Practice policies--guidelines for methods. JAMA 1990;263(13):1839-1841.

[23]   Eddy DM. Clinical decision making: from theory to practice. Guidelines for policy statements: the explicit approach. JAMA 1990;263(16):2239-40,2243.

[24]   Eddy DM. Comparing benefits and harms: the balance sheet. JAMA 1990;263(18):2493,2498,2501.

[25]   Mittman BS, Tonesk X, Jacobson PD. Implementing Clinical Practice Guidelines: Social Influence Strategies and Practitioner Behaviour Change. QRB Qual Rev Bull 1992;18(12):413-422.

[26]   Grol R. Implementing guidelines in general practice care. Quality in Health Care 1992;1:184-191.

[27]   Haines A, Jones R. Implementing findings of research. Br Med J 1994;308:1488-1493.

[28]   Wirtschafter D, Summers J, Jackson JR, Brooks CM, Turner M. Continuing medical educaiton using algorithms: a controlled trial assessment of effect of neonatal care. American Journal of Diseases of Childhood 1986;140:791-797.

[29]   Cohen DI, Littenberg B, Wetzel C, Neuhauser DB. Improving physician compliance with preventative medicine guidelines. Medical Care 1982;20:1040-1045.

[30]   Emslie CJ, Grimshaw J, Templeton A. Do clinical guidelines improve general practice management and referral of infertile couples? Br Med J 1993;306:1728-1731.

[31] Davidson RA, Fletcher SW, Retchie S, Duh S. A nurse intiated reminder system for the periodic health examination: implementation and evaluation. Arch Intern Med 1984;144:2167-2170.

[32] Sommers LS, Scholtz R, Shepherd RM, Starkweather DB. Physician involvement in quality assurance. Medical Care 1984;22:1115-1138.

[33] Tierney WM, Hui SL, McDonald CJ. Delayed feedback of physician performance versus immediate reminders to perform preventive care. Effects on physician compliance. Med Care 1986;24(8):659-666.

[34] Morgan M, Studney DR, Barnett GO, Winickoff RN. Computerized concurrent review of prenatal care. QRB Qual Rev Bull 1978;4:33-36.

[35] Chambers CV, Balaban DJ, Carlson BL, Ungemack JA, Grasberger DM. Microcomputer generated reminders. Improving the compliance of primary care physicians with mammography screening guidelines. J Fam Pract 1989;3:273-280.

[36] McAlister NH, Covvey DH, Tong C, Lee A, Wigle ED. Randomised controlled trial of computer assisted management of hypertension in primary care. Br Med J 1986;293:670-674.

[37] Thomas JC, Moore A, Qualls PE. The effect on cost of medical care for patients treated with an automated clinical audit system. Journal of Medical Systems 1983;7:307-313.

[38] Barnett GO, Winickoff R, Dorsey JL, Morgan M, Lurie RS. Quality assurance through automated monitoring and concurrent feedback using computer-based medical information system. Medical Care 1978;16:962-970.

[39] Barnett GO, Winickoff RN, Morgan MM, Zielstorff RD. A computer based monitoring system for follow-up of elevated blood pressure. Medical Care 1983;21:400-409.

[40] Brownridge G, Evans A, Fitter M, Platts M. An interactive computerised protocol for the management of hypertension: effects on the general practitioners clinical behaviour. J R Coll Gen Pract 1986;36:198-202.

[41] Evans AR, Wilkes ER, Absolon PJ, Denner TJ, Kaye G. An interactive computerised protocol for the management of hypertension. Methods Inf Med 1985;24:21-26.

[42] Margolis CZ, Warshawsky SS, Goldman L, Dagan O, Wirtschafter D, Pliskin JS. Computerized algorithms and pediatricians' management of common problems in a community clinic. Acad Med 1992;67(4):282-284.

[43] Petrucci K, Petrucci P, Canfield K, McComick KA, Kjerulff K, Parks P. Evaluation of UNIS: Urological Nursing Information System. Proc Annu Symp Comput Appl Med Care 1991;43-47.

[44] van der Lei J, van der Heijden P, Boon WM. Critiquing expert critiques: Issues for the development of computer-based monitoring in primary care. In: MEDINFO 89. (Eds: Barber,B; Cao,D; Qin,D; Wagner,G) North Holland Publ Comp, Amsterdam. 1989. 106-110.

[45] van der Lei J, van der Does E, Man in't Veld AJ, Musen MA, van Bemmel JH. Response of general practitioners to computer-generated critiques of hypertension therapy. Methods Inf Med 1993;32(2):146-153.

[46] Miller PL. ATTENDING: Critiquing a physcians management plan. IEEE Trans PAMI 1983;5:449-461.

[47] Lilford RJ, Kelly M, Baines A, Cameron S, Cave M, Gutherie K, et al. Effect of using protocols on medical care: randomised trial of three methods of taking an antenatal history. Br Med J 1992;305:1181-1184.

[48] Purves IN, Grimshaw JM. Computer generated protocols (letter). Br Med J 1993;306:460.

[49] Greenfield S, Lewis CE, Kaplan SH, Davidson MB. Peer review by criteria mapping: criteria for diabetes mellitus. The use of decision-making in chart audit. Ann Intern Med 1975;83(6):761-770.

[50] Margolis CZ. Uses of clinical algorithms. JAMA 1983;249:627.

[51] Grimm RH Jr, Shimoni K, Harlan WR Jr, Estes EH Jr. Evaluation of patient care protocol use by various providers. N Engl J Med 1975;292:507-511.

[52] Lomas J, Anderson GM, Domnick-Pierre K, Vayda E, Enkin MW, Hannah WJ. Do practice guidelines guide practice ? The effect of a consensus statement on the practice of physcians. N Engl J Med 1989;321:1311-1315.

[53] Shortliffe EH. Testing reality: the introduction of decision-support technologies for physicians. Methods Inf Med 1989;28(1):1-5.

[54] Komaroff AL. Algorithms and the 'Art of Medicine'. Am J Public Health 1982;72:10-12.

[55] Grol R. National standard setting for quality of care in general practice: attitudes of general practitioners and resonse to a set of standards. Br J Gen Pract 1990;40:361-364.

[56] Rosser W. Using perception-reality gap to alter prescribing patterns. J Med Educ 1983;57:722-761.

[57] Kassirer JP. Diagnostic Reasoning. Ann Intern Med 1989;110:893-900.

[58] Schmidt HG, Norman GR, Boshuizen HPA. A cognitive perspective on medical expertise: Theory and implications. Acad Med 1990;65(10):611-621.

[59] Style A. Intuition and problem solving. J R Coll Gen Pract 1979;29:71-74.

[60] Rogers EM. Diffusion of innovations. Free Press, New York. 1983.

[61] Dolan JG, Bordley DR. Using the analytic hierarchy process (AHP) to develop and disseminate guidelines. QRB Qual Rev Bull 1992;18(12):440-447.

[62] Field MJ, Lohr KN (Eds.). Guidelines for Clinical Practice: From Development to Use. National Academic Press, Washington,DC. 1992.

[63] Mold JW, Blake GH, Becker LA. Goal-oriented medical care. Fam Med 1991;23(1):46-51.

[64] Lomas J, Enkin M, Anderson GM, Hannah WJ, Vayda E, Singer J. Opinion leaders vs audit and feedback to implement practice guidelines. Delivery after previous caesarian section. JAMA 1991;265:2202-2207.

[65] Shiffman RN, Greenes RA. Rule set reduction using augmented decision table and semantic subsumption techniques: application to cholesterol guidelines. Proc Annu Symp Comput Appl Med Care 1992;339-343.

[66] Shiffman RN, Leape LL, Greenes RA. Translation of appropriateness criteria into practice guidelines: Application of decision table techniques to the RAND criteria for coronary artery bypass graft. Proc Annu Symp Comput Appl Med Care 1993;248-252.

[67] Quaak MJ, Westerman RF, van Bemmel JH. Comparisons between written and computerised patient histories. Br Med J 1987;295(6591):184-190.

[68] Coiera E. Questions and Assumptions. In: Knowledge and Decsions in Health Telematics. (Eds: Barahona,P; Christensen,JP) (Health Technology and Informatics: The next decade, 12.) IOS Press, Amsterdam. 1994. 61-66.

[69] Wyatt J. Promoting routine use of medical knowledge systems: Lessons from computerised ECG interpreters. In: Knowledge and Decsions in Health Telematics. (Eds: Barahona,P; Christensen,JP) (Health Technology and Informatics: The next decade, 12.) IOS Press, Amsterdam. 1994. 73-80.

[70] Timpka T, Nyce JM, Sjoberg C, Johansson M. Action design: from modelling to supprt of the software process. In: Proceedings of SEKE '92, San Fransisco. IEEE Press, Washington. 1993.

[71] Heathfield HA, Wyatt J. Philosophies for the design and developemnt of clinical decision support systems. Methods Inf Med 1993;32:1-8.

[72] Sackett DL. Rules of evidence and clinical recommendations on the use of antithrombotic agents. Chest 1986;86(2, Suppl.):2S-3S.

[73] Canadian Task Force on the Period Health Examination. The period health examination. Can Med Assoc J 1979;121:1193-1254.

[74] Acute pain management guideline panel (Ed.). Acute pain management: Operative or medical procedures and trauma. (92-0032) (Clinical Practice Guideline.) Agency for Health Care Policy and Research Publications, Rockville, MD. 1992.

[75] Lowe HJ, Barnett GO. Understanding and using the medical subject headings (MESH) vocabulary to perform literature searches. JAMA 1994;271(14):1103-1108.

[76] Lindberg DAB, Humphreys BL, McCray AT. The Unified Medical Language System. Methods Inf Med 1993;32(4):281-291.

[77] Eddy DM. Clinical decision making: from theory to practice. Connecting value and costs. Whom do we ask, and what do we ask them? JAMA 1990;264(13):1737-1739.

[78] Granneman T. Priority setting: A sensible approach to Medicaid policy? Inquiry 1991;28:300-305.

[79] Mayhew PJ, Dearney PA. An alternative prototyping classification. The Computer Journal 1987;30(6):481-484.

[80] Wyatt J, Spiegelhalter D. Evaluating medical expert systems: what to test and how? Med Inf (Lond) 1990;15(3):205-217.

[81] Martin J. Design and Construction. Vol. III. (Information Engineering.) Prentice Hall, Englewood Cliffs, NJ. 1990.

[82] McDonald C. Use of a computer to detect and respond to clinical events: Its effect on clinician behavior. Ann Intern Med 1976;84:162-167.

[83] McDonald CJ, Wilson GA, McCabe GP. Physician responses to computer reminders. JAMA 1980;244(14):1579-1581.

[84] Black N. Experimental and observational methods of evaluation (letter). Br Med J 1994;309:540.

[85] Sheldon TA. Please bypass the PORT. Br Med J 1994;309:142-143.

[86] Goldberg HI, Cummings MA, Steinberg EP, Ricci EM, Shannon T, Soumerai SB, Mittman BS, Eisenberg J, Heck DA, Kaplan S, et al. Deliberations on the dissemination of PORT products: translating research findings into improved patient outcomes. Med Care 1994;32(7, Suppl):JS90-J110.

[87] Kasper J, Mulley A, Wennberg J. Developing shared decision-making programs to improve the quality of health care. QRB Qual Rev Bull 1992;18:183-190.

[88] Wyatt J, Spiegelhalter D. Field trials of medical decision-aids: potential problems and solutions. Proc Annu Symp Comput Appl Med Care 1991;3-7.

[89] Booth NS, Purves IN. MIQUEST - A project to enable collection of morbidity data from different computer systems in primary care. In: Proceedings of MIE93. (Eds: Reichert,A; Sadan,BA; Bengtsson,S; Bryant,J; Piccolo,U) Freund Publishing House, London. 1993. 516-517.

[90] MIQUEST Project Team. MIQUEST Project Report. Version 3.3 ed. MIQUEST Project Board, Newcastle, UK. 1994.

[91] Markwell D. HQL: Express yourself and questions systems. Proceedings of the Annual Conference of the PHCSG of the BCS 1993;103-112.

[92] Hannah KJ, Conley-Price P, Fenty D, McKiel E, Soltes D, Hogan T, Wiens D. Computer applications for staff development and patient education. Methods Inf Med 1989;28:261-266.

[93] Mullins HC. Information technology in primary care. Proceedings of the Annual Conference of the PHCSG of the BCS 1993;4-11.

[94] Gagne RM, Briggs LJ. Principles of instructional design. 2nd ed. Holt, Rinehart and Winston, New York. 1979.

[95] Hripcsak G, Clayton P, Pryor A, Haug P, Wigertz O, van der Lei J. The Arden syntax for medical logic modules. Proc Annu Symp Comput Appl Med Care 1990;200-204.

[96] Gordon C, Herbert S I, Jackson-Smale A, Renaud-Salis J-L Care protocols and healthcare informatics Technology and informatics 10 - Artificial Intelligence in Medicine, IOS Press 289-309, 1993.

[97] Zander K. Critical pathways. Chap. 9. In: Total Quality Management: The Health Care Pioneers. (Eds: Melum,MM; Sinior,MK) American Hospital Publishing. 1992. pp. 305-314.

[98] Hofman PA. Critical path method: An important tool for co-ordinating clinical care. Journal on Quality Improvement 1993;19(7):235-246.

[99] DiJerome L. The nursing case management computerised system: Meeting the challenge of health care delivery through technology. Computers in Nursing 1992;10(6):250-258.

[100]Petryshen PR, Petryshen PM. The case management model: an innovative approach to the delivery of patient care. J Adv Nurs 1992;17:1188-1194.

[101]van der Lei J, Musen MA. A model for critiquing based on automated medical records. Comput Biomed Res 1991;24(4):344-378.

[102]Rucker DW, Shortliffe EH. A methodology for implementing clinical algorithms using expert-system and database tools. Proc Annu Symp Comput Appl Med Care 1989;33-37.

[103]Abendroth TW, Greenes RA, Joyce EA. Investigations in the use of clinical algorithms to organise medical knowledge. Proc Annu Symp Comput Appl Med Care 1988;90-95.

[104]Frisse ME. Searching for information in a hypertext medical handbook. Commun ACM 1988;31(7):880.

[105]Frisse ME. Retrieving Information From Medical Hypertext Systems. Proc Annu Symp Comput Appl Med Care 1988;441-444.

[106]Cimino JJ, Elkin PL, Barnett GO. As we may think: the concept space and medical hypertext. Comput Biomed Res 1992;25(3):238-263.

[107]Timpka T, Hedblom P, Tibblin G. A hypermedia document collection for primary care: why, what and how? Artif Intell Med 1990;2:179-192.

Knowledge engineering for drug prescribing guidelines

Robert Walton and Zeljko Ilic

ICRF General Practice Research Group, Department of Public Health and Primary Care, University of Oxford, Radcliffe Infirmary, Oxford OX2 6HE

Abstract. Prescribing drugs for the treatment of medical conditions is a very common activity for a doctor. Prescribing has enormous economic importance. Costs are rising quickly and there is an urgent need for doctors to have easy assess to advice about the cheapest, most effective therapy. On average 80% of GPs in the UK use a computer for their medical work and the figure is rising rapidly. Currently available systems provide only very simple checks and reminders. More sophisticated advice is provided by our prototype program. The program uses logic engineering to give advice, based on simple protocols for prescribing, tailored both to the condition being treated and the individual patient. The essential logical elements of the prescribing decision are discussed. These simple prescribing protocols may be the final common pathway for prescribing advice from many, more complex protocols for recommendations for drug treatment.

1 Introduction

Prescribing drugs is a common medical activity which takes place mainly in General Practice in the United Kingdom. A General Practitioner (GP) will generate about 60 prescriptions a day, each item costing about £8. The average practice prescribes 9508 items a year; the cost of these drugs is £278,656 for a single practice. [1] Drug costs are escalating rapidly and governments all over the European Union rightly wish to regulate prescribing. There is an urgent need for a computer system that can suggest safe, effective alternatives to high-cost drugs and thereby encourage rational prescribing.

In the United Kingdom incentives have recently been introduced to reduce the costs of prescribed drugs. GPs have been given a fund with which to buy medical care for their patients. "Fund holding" GPs will be able to use money that they save on drugs for other purposes such as employing extra staff. This financial "carrot" has made fund holders radically change their prescribing habits leading to a decrease in prescribing of expensive drugs. There has been a shift towards cheaper drugs that are just as effective. Non-fund holders are expected to take part in an incentive scheme to reduce their prescribing costs. This scheme has been less successful in reducing costs than the fund-saving option but nevertheless has helped to create a climate in which doctors are looking for drugs that are effective and cheap.

Overall 80% of practices in the United Kingdom (UK) are computerised although in some regions the figure is 94%. About 60% of GPs already use computers for prescribing.[2] Systems offering computer aided advice for prescribing in the United Kingdom are limited to warnings of drug interactions and GPs do not find them particularly useful. The systems warn GPs of interactions of which they are already aware and slow down the process of prescribing. In the DILEMMA project we are seeking to provide a much more comprehensive prescribing aid.[3] The system will have access to information already stored on the GP's computer about what drugs the patient has taken in the past and how well they worked for a particular condition. Information will also be available on how well the patient tolerated the drug in the past and whether there are any reasons why the drug should not be given such as other illnesses that the patient suffers from or other drugs he is already taking that interact. The system will contain recommendations for the best choice of drug for a particular condition and will give its advice tailored to the individual patient.

The system relies on a symbolic decision procedure [4] and uses logic programming techniques. This paper sets out the main factors that need to be taken into account when choosing a drug and outlines patient data, domain knowledge, and task knowledge for prescribing. We also examine the logical structure of the prescribing decision. The framework offers a way to encapsulate guidelines on what to do when a patient tolerates a drug poorly or the drug interacts with other drugs that the person is taking. These guidelines take input from our higher level guidelines for the management of asthma. The asthma protocol makes a general recommendation about which class of drug to use but relies on the prescribing guidelines to select the most appropriate drug and preparation for the individual patient.

2. Patient data model

Decision support for prescribing makes new demands of the basic patient record structure in the GP's computer. The decision to prescribe a drug is complex and this may explain why no systems are in common use in the UK despite high levels of computerisation.

2.1 Information about past use of a drug.

The doctor first needs to know if the patient has taken the drug in the past. This is important information since the safest option is always to give a drug that the patient has taken before and tolerated well.

In the DILEMMA project the basic structure of the patient record is:

```
patient_record(Date, Time, Code, PatientData ).
```

the information about past use of a drug is recorded:

```
patient_record(Date, Time, Code, (known(Drug))).
```

examples from our prototype system for prescribing for asthma:

```
patient_record(Date, Time, Code, (known(salbutamol)).
patient_record(Date, Time, Code, (known(terbutaline)).
patient_record(Date, Time, Code, (known(nedocromyl sodium)).
patient_record(Date, Time, Code, (known(ipratropium)).
```

2.2 Information about how well the patient tolerated the drug previously.

We consider that the information about how well the drug suited the patient can be broken down into four bands. The patient tolerates the drug well, has no side effects and feels quite happy with it:

```
patient_record(Date, Time,Code,(tolerates_well(ipratropium)).
```

If for example he does not like the taste or experiences some mild side effect but is happy to continue using the drug:

```
patient_record(Date, Time,Code,(tolerates(ipratropium)).
```

Similarly:

```
patient_record(Date, Time, Code,
(barely_tolerates(ipratropium)).patient_record(Date, Time, Code,
     (doesnt_tolerate(ipratropium)).
```

The latter case might indicate an allergy that was severe and meant that the patient should not take the drug again.

2.3 Information about whether the drug worked in the past.

Clearly whether the drug had the desired effect in the past is crucial information. The GP will usually ask "How well did it work last time you had it?" If the decision support system is to be as good or better than the GP it also needs to have this information available. We will need to persuade doctors that it is worthwhile taking the extra time to enter such data and this may be a problem with implementation.

Information concerning the efficacy of drugs may however already be available for some diseases from the practice computer. The severity of asthma is measured by the "peak expiratory flow rate" which is the velocity with which a patient can exhale measured in litres per minute. The GP's computer will have serial peak flow measurements over several years. If the GPs use their computers for prescribing the system could work out the average peak flow while taking a certain drug. Mathematical treatment of these data is possible in what has been called the "n of one " clinical trial. [5] This may be a useful method of determining with some precision how well a drug worked for a particular patient.

When the degree of efficacy has been determined the knowledge is represented thus:

```
patient_record(Date, Time, Code, (works(salbutamol,works)).
patient_record(Date, Time, Code, (works(terbutaline,works_well)).
patient_record(Date, Time, Code, (works(nedocromyl_sodium,works)).
```

3   Domain model.

The general way of representing medical knowledge in DILEMMA is:

```
domain(Object1, Relation, Object2).
```

For the prescribing task we have extended this representation to

```
domain(Object1, Relation, Object2, Strength).
```

Where Strength is a symbolic representative of the force of the relationship between the two objects.   Strength is one of {++,+,-,--}   depending upon the force of the relationship. Arguments with different forces can be combined according to the method of Huang et. al. [4]

3.1 Functional representation of domain knowledge.

We have developed a way of representing knowledge about a drug that is based on how the drug is used.

```
drugs(bronchodilator, has kind, beta agonist ).
drugs(bronchodilator, has kind, anticholinergic agent ).
drugs(beta agonist, has kind, short acting beta agonist ).
drugs(short acting beta agonist, has kind, terbutaline 100mcg inhaler).
drugs(short acting beta agonist, has kind, salbutamol 100mcg inhaler).
```

This functional classification has been used in our prototypes and found to be useful. The choice of representation was made after considering the two main sources of this information in common use in the United Kingdom, namely the Read Code Classification and the British National Formulary (BNF). The Read Code Classification is the most widely used by GP computer systems to store information about treatments and diseases.

Using the Read Codes hierarchy without modification would have resulted in:

```
drugs(respiratory drug, has kind, selective beta agonist).
drugs(selective beta agonist, has kind, salbutamol-inhalation preps).
drugs(salbutamol-inhalation preps, has kind, salbutamol 100mcg inhaler).
drugs(selective beta agonist, has kind, salbutamol-oral preparation).
```

but:

```
drugs(selective beta agonist, has kind, terbutaline sulphate resp).
drugs(terbutaline sulphate resp, has kind, terbutaline 500mcg inhaler).
```

so the information about the different types of preparations of terbutaline is stored at a higher level of the hierarchy.

and the British National Formulary:

```
drugs(respiratory drug, has kind, adrenoceptor stimulant).
drugs(adrenoceptor stimulant has kind, selective beta agonist).
drugs(selective beta agonist, has kind, salbutamol-oral preparation).
drugs(selective beta agonist, has kind, salbutamol-parenteral
preparation).
drugs(selective beta agonist, has kind, salbutamol-inhalation preps).
drugs(salbutamol-inhalation preps, has kind, salbutamol 100mcg inhaler).
```

Here the information is stored at the same level of the hierarchy for both salbutamol and terbutaline. However neither of the two systems in common use make the distinction between long acting and short acting beta agonists which is necessary for reasoning about how to use the drug in asthma. It may be necessary to adapt an existing classification specifically for decision support so that we can develop a logical functional classification.

Our knowledge of diseases in which a drug should not be used is based on that supplied by Exeter Database Systems (EDBS). The EDBS system specifies only 50 disease types in which certain drugs should not be used. We have mapped Read Codes onto these EDBS codes so that each EDBS "parent" has several Read "children."

```
prescribing(Formulation, not used with, EDBSdisease, Strength).
prescribing(naproxen 500mg tabs, not used with, duodenal ulcer, +).

prescribing(EDBSdisease, has kinds, Readdisease).
prescribing(duodenal ulcer, has kinds, duodenal ulcer anterior).
prescribing(duodenal ulcer, has kinds, duodenal ulcer posterior).
prescribing(duodenal ulcer, has kinds, perforated duodenal ulcer).
```

and so on. A similar mapping is used for drug interactions.

Drug combinations

Many drugs are prescribed in combination for the treatment of particular diseases. In the treatment of cancer, cyclophosphamide, methotrexate and 5-fluorouracil may be prescribed with an antiemetic. If the antiemetic were not used the patient would suffer unacceptable nausea. Our prototype treats drug combinations as single structured objects:

```
drug_combination(1, [cyclophosphamide, methotrexate, 5-flourouracil,
metoclopramide]).
```

Attributes belong to the structured object and not its component parts.

```
patient_record(Date, Time, Code, tolerates([cyclophosphamide,
methotrexate, 5-flourouracil, metoclopramide])).
```

and the following may also be true:

```
patient_record(Date, Time, Code, (doesnt tolerate([cyclophosphamide,
methotrexate, 5-flourouracil]))).
```

Drug combinations are treated similarly in the argumentation procedure described later.

Drug dosages.

The prototype has very simple rules to suggest dosages based on age:

```
dosage( `trimethoprim`, Age, Dosage) :- Age > 0.17, Age =< 0.42,
      Dosage = `25mg every 12 hours`.
dosage( `trimethoprim`, Age, Dosage) :- Age > 0.42, Age =< 5,
      Dosage = `50mg every 12 hours`.
dosage( `trimethoprim`, Age, Dosage) :- Age > 5, Age =< 12,
      Dosage = `100mg every 12 hours`.
dosage( `trimethoprim`, Age, Dosage) :- Age > 12,
      Dosage = `200mg every 12 hours`.
```

3.1 Formulary.

The formulary is a large knowledge base containing drugs linked to the diseases that they treat. The knowledge base also contains the strength of the recommendation for treatment and reflects the practice formulary agreed by the general practitioners in our trial practice.

So for example:

```
prescribing(antibiotic, has kinds, flucloxacillin 250mg tabs).
prescribing(flucloxacillin 250 mg tabs, treats, skin infection, +).
```

Flucloxacillin is the antibiotic used most frequently for infections of the skin (Table 2). This is because infections are usually caused by staphylococcus which is often resistant to penicillin. Where we know the underlying medical reasons for the decision (Table 1) we reason with it thus:

```
prescribing(staphylococcus, causes, skin infection, +).
prescribing(flucloxacillin 250mg caps, treats, staphylococcus, +)
prescribing(penicillin 250mg tabs, treats, staphylococcus, -)
prescribing(erythromycin 250mg tabs, treats, staphylococcus, +)
prescribing(trimethoprim 200mg tabs, treats, staphylococcus, +)
```

Weighting different kinds of evidence in prescribing.

The weighting of the recommendations in the prototype depends upon expert opinion. This opinion will take into account many different kinds of evidence. Table 1 gives the types of evidence ranked according to the weight that experts give to it.

An experiment on one person otherwise called the "n of one " controlled trial is the strongest argument for prescribing a particular drug. With this technique a drug is used for a period of time and the response of some indicator of the disease is monitored. The change in the indicator is compared statistically with placebo in a double blind fashion. Experiments such as these are rarely carried out in General Practice and they are only suitable for chronic diseases. However it may be that in the future computer prescribing systems will facilitate these trials.

Randomised controlled trials (RCTs) are the main form of evidence used to assess the worth of a particular treatment for a disease. Statistical methods already exist for aggregating data from different trials into meta-analyses. Where meta-analyses exist they are the next strongest reason for using a particular treatment. RCTs are expensive to conduct and so have not been performed for the bulk of problems encountered in General Practice. Necessarily RCTs have rigorous entry criteria and patients are excluded on grounds such as age or sex. The GP often then cannot extrapolate the results of a published trial directly to his/her patient.

Table 1

Weighting evidence for prescribing

---

1. Scientific experiment on an individual
    -"n of one " controlled trial

2. Population based data
    -meta-analyses
    -single randomised controlled trial
    -cohort studies
    -case control
    -epidemiological studies

3. Peer aided judgement
    -Consensus Statements
    -Guidelines
    -Protocols
    -Practice formulary

4. Case reports

5. Anecdotal

Many prescribing decisions in General Practice are made on the basis of recommendations of groups of experts making decisions about treatments. Different groups of experts may come to different conclusions and the GP may be faced with a difficult task resolving these problems. More general statements of policy are published in reference books such as the British National Formulary. Each general practice produces its own formulary of diseases and treatments which is usually a subset of the British National Formulary and reflects the individual opinions of the GPs.

There are no formal methods of aggregating data from different categories such as case reports and meta-analyses. It may be that in the future the DSS will be able to assess the weight of evidence and make recommendations using symbolic methods of argumentation.

4 Task model.

The task model used in the DILEMMA project allows the knowledge author to define the force of arguments for the prescribing task.

```
task(Role, Task, Relation).
```

Where Role identifies how the argument is used in the reasoning procedure:

```
Role ∈{proposing,refining,excluding,confirming,supporting,diminishing}.
```
or
```
Role ∈{proposing,refining,--,++,+,-,  }.
```

A diminishing argument in prescribing would be that a drug had a high cost:

```
task(diminishing, prescribing, high cost).
```

An excluding argument might be:

```
task(excluding, prescribing, age<16).
```

meaning that the drug should not be used for children. For this particular task, it is possible to refine the supporting and diminishing arguments further. To do this we need to examine the way the decision is structured.

4.11 The logical structure of the prescribing decision.

We consider the structure of the decision to be a simple balance of the arguments for and against using a particular drug for a disease shown in Table 2.

Supporting Arguments.

There are two main arguments in favour of using a drug. The first comes from a consideration of how much benefit the patient will gain from taking the drug. This is the

Table 2

The Prescribing decision

Arguments for using a drug	*Arguments Against*
1. Strength of Recommendation	1. Contraindications
2. Past experience of the drug	2. Interactions
-previous use	3. Cost
-previous efficacy	
-previous level of tolerance	

---

strength of the recommendation and derived largely, in our prototype, from expert opinion. The second major argument depends upon how effective and how well tolerated the drug was in the past. This information is gained from the patient record on the GPs computer. These two arguments are given equal weight in the decision procedure.

Diminishing Arguments.

There are three main arguments against using the drug. The patient may have some pre-existing disease which would make it dangerous or disadvantageous to use the drug. In this case the drug is said to be contraindicated.

```
prescribing(naproxen 500mg tabs,not used with, duodenal ulcer, -).
```

If however the patient is taking a drug which interacts with the new drug then it may be more sensible not to start the new treatment. These interactions are rarely absolute and their force is recorded in the usual way.

```
prescribing(naproxen 500mg tabs, interacts with, warfarin 3mg tabs, - ).
```

The interaction between warfarin and naproxen does not usually cause problems if the dose of warfarin is monitored carefully.

The final consideration is the cost of the drug. Making rational decisions about the cost of drug is difficult because drugs are often used in different doses for different illnesses. Also different drugs of the same class may not be equally potent. Comparison between drugs has been facilitated by the World Health Organisation concept of a "defined daily dose." (WHO 93) This the total amount of the drug that is usually taken each day.

Because costs for defined daily doses are not available in electronic format we have used data from Exeter Database Systems Philex database data to approximate them for the prototype.

```
prescribing(naproxen 500mg tabs, costs, - ).
```

The decision procedure gives equal weight to these three arguments against using the drug.

The final result is produced by reasoning with the arguments for and against each candidate. The candidates are presented to the user in the rank order in which they were supported.

Resolving conflict between tolerance and efficacy.

The balance of how well tolerated the drug was against its effectiveness is not simple.

We need to reason with information on tolerance and efficacy to decide for the individual patient what the preferred treatment is. To do this we use a constrained decision procedure shown in Table 3.

Table 3. Balancing tolerance and efficacy

	tolerates well	tolerates	barely tolerates	does not tolerate
works well	1200	1100	800	0
works	1100	1000	600	0
barely works	500	200	100	0
does not work	0	0	0	0

Each combination is assigned a rating which was determined empirically. The ratings will be "fine tuned" with further use. The procedure gives greater weight to a drug that was poorly tolerated yet still worked. This procedure can be seen as a specific instance of the more general DILEMMA argumentation procedure described elsewhere. (4)

We represent this as:

```
rating(tolerates_well, works_well, 1200).
rating(tolerates_well, works,1100).
rating(tolerates_well, barely_works, 500).
```

and so on.

If the patient has not taken the drug before the rating is set at 600.

Eventually data will accumulate on the system concerning the tolerance and efficacy of particular drugs in the population as a whole. This valuable data will allow the DSS to propose a new drug in a particular patient. The system would check past records of treatments for an illness and select the most appropriate treatment.

Co-existing diseases.

It is often the case that two diseases are present at the same time. Returning to our previous example of antibiotic prescribing in section 3.1. Consider the problem of a patient who has both a skin and a chest infection. In this case the system will recommend the antibiotic effective against both.

```
prescribing(pneumococcus, causes, chest infection, +).
prescribing(haemophilus influenzae, causes, chest infection, +).
prescribing(staphylococcus, causes, chest infection, -)
prescribing(trimethoprim 200mg tabs, treats, haemophilus influenzae, +)
prescribing(trimethoprim 200mg tabs, treats, pneumococcus , +)
```

The DSS would suggest that trimethoprim is the most appropriate antibiotic because it treats pneumococcus and haemophilus which can cause chest infections and also the staphylococcus which causes the skin infection.

5 Conclusion.

We have demonstrated how important a task prescribing is in medical practice and highlighted the need to reduce costs and improve quality. We believe that computer decision support systems have an important part to play in this and suitable hardware is already available on GPs desks. Decision support will place new demands on the patient record information stored on GP computers and we have sought to highlight the areas where improvement is needed.

Existing classifications and taxonomies are not designed for decision support and we have considered outlines of a logical functional classification for drugs. Our prototypes however make full use of existing knowledge bases where possible.

The structure of the prescribing decision is complex and we have provided a model for it which has been used in the prototype decision support system. This model follows the same principles of argumentation as that produced earlier in the DILEMMA project but allows further refinement of supporting and diminishing arguments for choosing drugs. The structure suggested allows the knowledge contained in simple prescribing guidelines to be translated into a form with which machines can reason to provide decision support.

References

[1] Anon. PACT Report 1993 Sept-Dec. In: Prescription Pricing Authority, PO Box 1YG. Newcastle upon Tyne. NE99 1YG, 1993:

[2] Social Surveys (Gallup Poll) Limited. Computerisation in GP Practices 1993 Survey. Department of Health (Management Executive), 1993:40.

[3] Gordon C. Dilemma: Logic Engineering in General Practice, Oncology and Shared Care. AIM 1992 Telematics Systems in Health Care 1992;(5):22-25.

[4] Huang J, Fox J, Gordon C, Jackson-Smale A. Symbolic Decision Support in Medical Care. Artificial Intelligence in Medicine 1993;5:415-430.

[5] Guyatt H, Sackett D, Taylor DW. Determining optimal therapy-randomised trials in individual patients. N. Engl. J. Med. 1986;314:889.

Computerized Assessment with Primary Care Guidelines in the Netherlands

P.E. Zanstra and W.P.A. Beckers

Dept. Medical Informatics, Epidemiology & Statistics, POB 9101, NL-6500 HB N ijmegen,
The Netherlands

Abstract. To promote quality assurance and expertise in primary health care in the Netherlands the Dutch College of General Practitioners develops protocols, called standards. These standards concern medical action-taking in case of regular complaints and diseases in common practice. To improve dissemination of the standards and to develop effective and useful methods for quality assurance on the basis of the standards a project, called the Guidelines Automation Project (Richtlijnen Automatiseringsproject) was started to develop a computer program that can support quality assurance of medical action-taking in general practice on the basis of the NHG-standards. The main feature of the program is educational assessment. Other features of the program are: guidance for case data collection, stating of differential diagnoses, and disease profiles. These features also use patient case data as a starting point. In conclusion it is argued that all efforts towards an 'electronic' use of protocols in the health care delivery system will fail, unless we arrive at a care record that both with respect to its structure and to its content, is being founded on sound formal principles. Several problems need to be solved first. The implementation, and exploitation of protocols, though relatively simple from a knowledge representation point of view, is not a straightforward task.

1 Introduction

In primary health care in the Netherlands, the need for quality assurance and expertise improvement has led to the development of Guidelines. These Guidelines, called standards, are part of a system of regular and structured quality assurance and quality improvement for general practitioners. The Dutch College of General Practitioners (NHG) formulated these standards on the basis of recent scientific insights and in collaboration with specialists in specific fields. Where scientific research concerning a certain subject was inadequate, consensus procedures were carried out. These NHG standards have a country-wide validity. Support in practical situations, prevention of unjustified diversity in medical action-taking, and consolidation of the general practitioners' professional status are the main objectives of the standards. The broadly based acceptance of standards is on itself no guarantee that GPs work in accordance with these standards. Even if one knows what ideally must be done in a specific situation, such information does not suffice to create correspondingly adapted individual practice routines (1). Therefore the main question is to disseminate the standards in such a way that GPs are willing to adjust their working methods to these standards. Quality assurance and expertise enhancement in medicine will benefit from immediate feedback in practice, especially when this feedback fits in the practitioners' own procedures (2,3). The need for fast feedback becomes even more relevant since the number of standards is rapidly growing. In general practice vocational training and assessment will benefit from feedback to elucidate differences between GPs. Mostly, this gives strong impulses to critical reflection on individual working methods (4-7).

To improve dissemination of the standards and to develop effective and useful methods for quality assurance on the basis of the standards, a project, called the Guidelines Automation Project (Richtlijnen Automatiseringsproject) was started to develop a computer program that can support quality assurance of medical action taking in general practice on the basis of the NHG standards. The program provides two functions:

- Education:
    transfer of Guidelines. For training of students and refresher courses for GPs, relevant history-taking and sample patient cases are added.
- Evaluation and Assessment:
    - evaluation of student GPs (external assessment): on the basis of standardised situations or real patient cases assessment will take place. The program provides feedback about progress and gaps and allows for comparison between trainees;
    - self-assessment: individual GPs are able to enter their actions concerning individual patients and will be provided with feedback;
    - assessment of GPs in continuing medical education: groups of GPs are able to enter their actions concerning series of patients with similar complaints or diseases and are provided with feedback and differences related to one another.

The Quality Assurance in Primary Care project was divided in two main phases. The first phase consisted of two activities. First the guidelines had to be transformed into an audit instrument. This appeared not to be as easy as it looked on first sight. The individual guidelines were developed by different groups. Moreover the development work was paper-based. It was found that the guidelines had internal inconsistencies, but also there were inconsistencies between the different standards. After this first activity was ended, the guidelines automation project (RAP) started with the computer implementation of the guidelines themselves, and the auditing strategies. The second phase comprised the comparison of the effectiveness of different auditing methods, such as the computer-based audit versus a paper-based audit. The other activity in the second phase was the large scale (500 GPs) introduction of the audit program. The whole project was supported by organizations including professional bodies, the Ministry of Health, insurance companies.

In this presentation we will focus on the computer implementation RAP.

2 The RAP program

The intended use of the program was as stated above in quality assurance, but it also was intended to be an instrument in enhancement of skills, and for use in vocational training. We decided to have an initial trial phase to prove the validity of the concept. We therefore set up a pilot study with eight GPs. The RAP program was implemented on the basis of the Relation Oriented Inference System (ROIS) (8). There were a number of prerequisites set out for the program:

- The program must be PC based, simple and intuitive to use, also for the novice user.
- The program should run on simple 286 machines which still were predominantly the type of equipment in use by the profession.
- The program should deliver quick feedback about the course of action in a specific case.

- The program should be able to produce 'aggregated' feedback about the user's performance in a broader scope of medical action taking.
- The program must have added value with respect to the current audit practice
- The program must be able to instantly support the course of action in an advisory setting.

The NHG standards make up the domain of the knowledge bases in the RAP program. The RAP program currently facilitates:
- case creation and case modification;
- (self-)assessment concerning one single case, including explanation;
- (self-)assessment for all cases concerning a single standard;
- (self-)assessment for all cases concerning multiple standards.

2.1 Case creation and case modification

Part of the RAP program is a database where patient cases can be stored. One of the programs' facilities is to create new cases and to modify existing ones.

Guided by the program creation of a new case starts by selecting one of the NHG standards from the domain. Subsequently all possible actions and related results are shown, from which performed actions and facts observed can be marked. All marked items including the selected NHG standard will be stored in the patient case file.

Updating of an existing patient case uses the same facility. Here however there is no prompting to select a NHG standard as it is already present in the case file. Only actions and related results are shown that are not present in the case file yet. Removal of items from the case file is also supported by the program.

2.2 Self-assessment concerning one single case

For assessment concerning one single case the particular case must be selected. Execution of the task Assessment generates feedback concerning the selected case by matching the case items with the related NHG standard.

The program shows feedback considering all case items. Feedback is given in three parts:

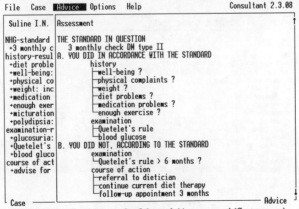

Figure 1 : Feedback as result of the task 'Assessment' (first screen).

- what has been done in accordance with the standard;
- what has been not done although recommended by the standard;
- what has superfluously been done.

Depending on the standard feedback may fill more screens. The user can scroll through the whole feedback, which in this case is three screens. For assessment concerning one single case the particular case must be selected. Execution of the task Assessment generates feedback concerning the selected case by matching the case items with the corresponding NHG standard. Depending on the guidelines stated in the standard, the program determines whether the case items matches the prescribed actions and the appropriateness of their sequence. The system's response for the specimen case 'Suline I.N.' is shown in Figures 1-3.

2.3 Self-assessment for all cases concerning one single standard

The program offers a facility to aggregate assessment results concerning one particular NHG standard. The task 'Aggregation of one standard' searches the database for all matching patient cases and aggregates all feedback items.

The program shows feedback considering all case items. Feedback is given in five parts:
- the actual standard, between brackets the number of cases concerning that standard (Fig. 4);
- in accordance with the standard (Fig. 4);
- not done although recommended by the standard (Fig. 5);
- superfluously been done (partially in Fig. 5);
- actions that don't belong to the standard (not shown).

Depending on the standard feedback may fill more screens. The user can scroll through the whole feedback, which in this case is two screens.

2.4 Self-assessment for all cases concerning multiple standards

The program offers a facility to aggregate assessment results concerning more than one particular NHG standard. The task 'Aggregation of more standards' searches the database for all matching patient cases and aggregates all feedback items.

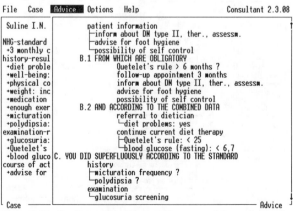

Figure 2: Feedback as result of the task 'Assessment' (second screen).

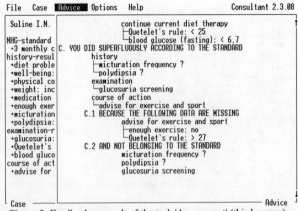

Figure 3: Feedback as result of the task 'Assessment' (third screen).

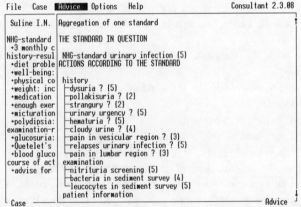

Figure 4: Feedback as result of the task 'Aggregation of one standard' (first screen).

```
 File   Case  Advice  Options   Help                Consultant 2.3.08

 Suline I.N. │ ACTIONS THAT SHOULD HAVE BEEN DONE                      ↑
             │
 NHG-standard│ history
  +3 monthly c│  ┌pollakisuria ? (3)
 history-resul│  ├strangury ? (3)
  +diet proble│  ├cloudy urine ? (1)
  +well-being:│  ├pain in vesicular region ? (2)
  +physical co│  ├pain in lumbar region ? (2)
  +weight: inc│  └persisting mictur. compl. after therapy? (1)
  +medication │ examination
  +enough exer│  ┌bacteria in sediment survey (1)
  +micturation│  ├recurrent nitrituria survey (3)
  +polydipsia:│  ├check examination bacteria in sediment (1)
 examination-r│  └check examination leucocytes in sediment (1)
  +glucosuria:│ patient information
  +Quetelet's │  ┌complete bladder emptying (4)
  +blood gluco│  └drinking enough (4)
 course of act│ course of action
  +advise for │  └urinary infection profylaxis (2)
             │ ACTIONS THAT HAVE SUPERFLUOUSLY BEEN DONE
             │
             │  examination
 └ Case ──────┴───────────────────────────────────────── Advice ┘
```

Figure 5: Feedback as result of the task 'Aggregation of one standard' (second screen)

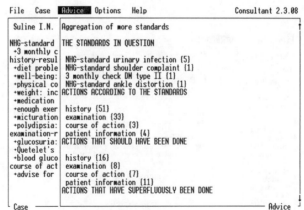

Figure 6: Feedback as result of the task 'Aggregation of more standards (only first screen shown).

As actions differ from standard to standard, feedback only concerns the consultation phase in which these actions were performed. The program shows feedback considering all case items per consultation phase. Feedback is given infive parts:
- the actual standards, beeen brackets the number of cases concerning each particular standard;
- in accordance with the standards, between brackets the number of these actions per consultation phase;
- not done although recommended by the standards;
- superfluously done;
- actions that don't belong to the standards.

Depending on the standard feedback may fill more screens. The user can scroll through the whole feedback, which in this case is one screen (Figure 6)

In addition to the aggregation of performance of the individual, in one of the experiments also an aggregation over the group as a whole was made. This was not done with the RAP program, but by separate analysis. The basic data however were extracted from usage log files produced by the RAP program. In this feedback the individual user was shown how his performance was with respect to the performance of his (peer review) group. From the questionnaires sent out in the evaluation, it appeared that this kind of feedback, and the aggregation of performance with respect to all standards was the most appreciated feedback. The reasons for that have not been fully cleared yet, but certainly one of the elements is that one never encounters a prototypical patient, to whom the specific protocol applies. Doctors had the feeling that the individual cases considered in the audit were not always fully covered by the protocol. They deliberately had to deviate from the standard. However the more abstract aggregations gave them feedback in terms of ' being not very strong in patient education', but 'quite good at medical action taking' (cf. Fig. 7).

2.5 Enhanced facilities of the RAP program

The starting point of the RAP program was its use as a tool for educational self-assessment. It was not aimed at supporting selective assessment, as for example in the context of recertification. The facilities of the semantic network processor ROIS however, enables the

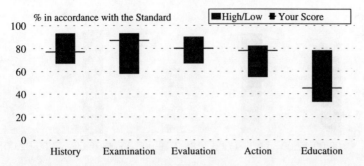

Figure 7: As part of one of the experiments, also the performance of the whole testgroup of 26 GPs was reported back to the individual GP. The high and low scores of the group in treatment of 'soar throat' are plotted with as a horizontal line the performance of the individual GP.

implementation of more inference tasks that make use of the same knowledge base (9). Additional inferences were designed for the following tasks:

- Advice: the GP may use the program to get advice on the next step during consultation considering the already known patient data;
- Disease Profile: the program shows all diseases (if any) covered by the standard corresponding to the patient case at hand;
- Differential Diagnosis: the program shows all possible diagnosis from the standard concerning the case at hand. From each disease the present and the missing data are listed. The disease that is completely consistent with the patient's data is mentioned.

3 Evaluation of the RAP program

The RAP program was evaluated by twenty six general practitioners. The evaluation consisted of automatic registration of assessment results and an evaluation form. The evaluation form showed that:

- the programs' clarity, unambiguousness and user-friendliness were assessed as being clearly sufficient;
- feedback (assessment and aggregation) was at the first glance found complicated, but became quite understandable after working with the program;
- individual well-reasoned deviation from the standards is not supported by the program;
- computerised assessment is a convenient method to get acquainted with and work along the lines of the NHG standards.
- The program was hardly used during patient encounters (cf. Figure 8.)

After being successfully evaluated in a field trial with some 50 GPs, the program is now being distributed to 500 GPs in the Guidelines Implementation Project (RIP).

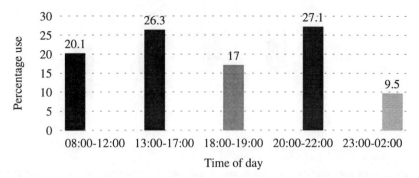

Figure 8: Usage of the system. This figure shows the percentage of use of the program in one of the pilots. It was relatively little used during patient encounter times of day (8-12 am).

4 Preliminary conclusions

Although the RAP program was evaluated as satisfactory with respect to the requirements (see par 2.), the current use in the RIP project is disappointingly low. This result did not come as a complete surprise. After a very successful evaluation (10) of the Internist system as a 'clinical advisor' it never became widely used like that. It rather evolved into an electronic intelligent book. It was rather cumbersome to enter all medical facts, which made it only useful for specific occasions. Entering facts about a patient was not a problem in RAP. The system is very quick. However in the current age of fancy coloured windows the ROIS user interface looks old-fashioned. This is partially a reason for not using the system. We think however there are more important grounds for this apparent failure. The inability of (knowledge based) systems to sensibly connect to the health care record is in our view a major obstacle for further dissemination of the program.

- There is a lack of common 'standardised' medical language to fully and unambiguously describe the patient's health status.
- There is a lack of a common 'standardised' structure for registering patient data.

In fact we believe that all efforts towards an 'electronic' use of protocols in the health care delivery system will fail, unless we arrive at a care record that both with respect to its structure and to its content, is being founded on sound formal principles. Within the EU-AIM framework, the GALEN project holds the promise to serve as the 'lingua franca' to tackle the first problem. Several projects see this as a sensible solution. With respect to the structure of the health care record there is a greater diversity in visions. A unified view seems still to be far away.

So though protocols because of several reasons (see Barahona's chapter this book on the recommendations of the Epistol action) may seem an obvious target for further exploitation, we would strongly advise that the implementation and exploitation of protocols, despite their relative representational simplicity, is not a straightforward task!

Acknowledgement

This research was partially funded by the Dutch Ministry of Public Health, and through the EU-AIM projects Dilemma and Galen. The co-operation with the Centre of Quality Assurance Research of the Universities of Nijmegen and Limburg in the RAP projects is kindly acknowledged.

References

[1] Sanazaro, P. Determining physicians performance. Evaluation and Health Professions 1983; 2: 197-210.
[2] Lomas, J., Anderson, G.M., Domnick-Pierre, K., Vayda, E., Enkin and M.W., Hannah, W.J. (1989) Do practice guidelines guide practice? The effect of consensus statement on the practice of physicians. NEJM, 19:1306-1311.
[3] Sheldon, M. (1983) Microcomputers in medical audit and continuing education. Update,26:463-469.
[4] Grol, R.P.T.M. (1990) National standard setting for quality of care in general practice: attitudes of general practitioners and response to a set of standards. BJGP, 40:361-364.
[5] Forrest, J., Mc Kenna, M., Stanley, I. (1989) Continuing education: a survey among general practitioners. FP, 6:98-107.
[6] Owen, P., Allery, L., Hardny, K., Hays, T. (1989) General practitioners' continuing medical education within and outside their practice. BMJ, 299:238-240
[7] Bloemer, J., Poiesz, T. (1987) Nascholingsbehoeften en -wensen bij de Nederlandse huisarts. Verslag van een consumentenonderzoek. Tilburg: Katholieke Universiteit Brabant.
[8] Vries Robbé, P.F. de, Zanstra, P.E., Beckers, W.P.A. (1989) Relation Oriented Inference System (ROIS). In: Proc. AIT 89. Herik, H.J. van der. (Ed.) Amsterdam: SIC,:317-325.
[9] Vries Robbé, P.F. de, Zanstra, P.E., Hartkamp, S.F., Beckers, W.P.A. (1989) MEDES as a tool for different reasoning strategies. In: Proc. AIME 89. Hunter, J., Cookson, J., Wyatt, J. (Eds.), London: Springer Verlag,:309-315.
[10] Miller, R.A., Pople, H.E., Myers, M.D. (1982) Internist-I, an experimental computer-based diagnostic consultant for general internal medicine, NEJM 307 pp 468-476.

Health Telematics for Clinical Guidelines and Protocols
C. Gordon and J.P. Christensen (Eds.)
IOS Press, 1995

Primary Care Guidelines from an organizational point of view

A.J. ten Hoopen, D.A. Boon, J. Nutma and P.F. de Vries Robbé

Dept. Medical Informatics, Epidemiology & Statistics, University of Nijmegen
P.O. Box 9101, 6500 HB Nijmegen, The Netherlands

Abstract. Guidelines in primary health care have been developed to reduce assumed and undesired variation in certain aspects of care delivery by professionals. If systematically applied guidelines no doubt effect the quality of care. It is argued however that taking an organizational point of view on quality management yields new requirements with respect to development and application of guidelines. It is considered to be essential for managerial control purposes that guidelines have simple and valid indicators to monitor the actual application and to measure the preferred outcome. It is essential that the choice of guidelines to be implemented in an organization is determined in the context of an explicit plan for quality management.

1 Introduction

For quality management in primary health care (PHC) in the Netherlands the dominant role is played by the Guidelines developed by the Dutch College of General Practitioners [1]. The set of guidelines emerged incrementally from the start in 1989 with a handful of guidelines dealing with conditions or problems where undesirable variation in handling by Dutch GP's was to be reduced. The current set of over 40 guidelines is the result of a policy of the College [2] based on scientific evidence and the opinions of various groups in the Dutch society. It is definitely not the exclusive result of a systematic analysis of the complete set of health problems presented [3,4], of variation in behaviour of GP's [4] and its causes, or of the possibilities for influencing those causes by the introduction of guidelines.

Apart from the guidelines for GPs developed by the College there are at least two other PHC-areas where guideline development has relevance for PHC organizations.

On the one hand there are the guidelines developed by GP's and pharmacists [5] to rationalize the prescription and delivery of drugs in PHC, i.e. to banish all kinds of undesired variation in prescribing for a given condition, and, through generic prescribing, to control the cost of drugs actually delivered.

On the other hand Centres for PHC in the Netherlands have traditionally since their origination in the early seventies focussed on coordination of care delivery and cooperation of different disciplines dealing with the same patient/problem: shared care. These Centres for PHC with their organizational overhead have always had an urge to prove their surplus value to financing institutions.

They have, therefore, embodied their policies in guidelines [6]. These deal with the following topics: multiple problems of elderly, sleeping problems, arthrosis, urinary incontinence of elderly women, diabetes mellitus type II, stress complaints, low back pain, homecare for the terminal ill, CNSLD in children, policies on prescription and delivery of drugs.

Both developments share with the development of GP guidelines their establishment through a consensus procedure and the rather arbitrary composition of the set of guidelines.

In the contribution of Zanstra et al. in this book [7] the goal of the RAP program is summed up as the possibility to make statements on three levels:

- the way an individual case of a problem or disease type has been dealt with given the characteristics of the case (the individual patient level in evaluations)

- the way a problem or disease type has been dealt with (the single guideline level)

- the way GP's perform procedures that may be part of different guidelines (the level of technical procedure performance).

These requirements of the RAP program emerge from an analysis of needs for support of the quality assurance activities of GP's. This analysis however is restricted to evaluations of the use of *available* guidelines, which is, due to the lack of a unifying meta guideline, of course a too narrow vision on what the quality management process in general practice or the whole of PHC is about. Missing in the analysis is for example the level of the complete work and output as performed by a GP or even wider of PHC organisations. To put it in other words: there is not yet a clearly demarcated picture of a process with an associated product in which the use of guidelines is embedded. This descriptive process definition is needed in order to define the management of quality for this process.

The aim of this contribution is to try to use process modelling techniques from information systems development and concepts of quality management to make the additional requirements for primary care guidelines explicit if one takes the viewpoint of a manager responsible for a whole PHC organization.

2. Quality management in Centres for PHC

Dealing with the development of information services in Centres for PHC [8] *including* the support of management, the authors have tried to apply some basic assumptions. Firstly, to perform adequately any activity in an organisation, be it delivery of care by a professional or quality control by managers for example, one has to *have available the information needed* for that activity. And not just available, but in time, correctly, completely, aggregated as needed etc. Secondly, to determine what information is needed for complex activities connected to diagnosing and treating health problems including managerial control of health care delivery one has to use a *descriptive model* of every activity to synthesize the information needs [9]. Thirdly one has to distinguish explicitly between *primary activities* and *management* of those activities. Management after all has (we assume!) its own specific information needs which require recording of data by primary activities that are not directly needed by those activities themselves. For example it is often of no use to the GP for the treatment of a patient to record that certain steps from a protocol are applied. But it is definitely of use to do so for the quality manager to be able to count for example the number of times in a given period and for certain patient classes (part of) a protocol has been applied. Fourthly, quality management has to be done by every organization in health care, be it a single handed GP cooperating with the local physiotherapist and/or community nurse, or a Centre for PHC housing a group practice of ten GP's together with other kinds of PHC professionals working together. And they all lack time to do a thorough analysis on how to deal with the problems of establishing an adequate information service for quality management.

So it is valuable to describe the primary and (quality) management processes in a generic way, independent of the specific combinations of tasks and responsibilities in jobs in organizations.

Starting from these basic assumptions, a reference business and information model has been developed for the processes of Centres for PHC in the Netherlands [8]. This reference information model also addresses quality management at both strategic management and managerial control level.

The overall business model is outlined in figure 1.

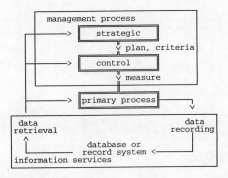

Figure 1. Overview of the processes

Figure 1 gives the main decomposition in processes and basic information & data flow, while in figure 2 (below) the generic structure of the primary processes contained in the overall process model for every PHC function is described. In PHC centres in the Netherlands one typically finds several of the following primary, supporting and management processes:

Table A. Names of processes distinguished in Centres for PHC.

general medical care	nursing & home help	psychological & social services
pharmaceutical care	physiotherapy	midwifery
dental care	dietetics	shared care
public health care		
appointment coordination	patient registration	financial affairs
resource management	production management	quality management
general policymaking		

On the basis of the generic process model for health care delivery in figure 2, which resulted from a study of the literature and job or task descriptions in several Centres, information needs have been determined in interviews with professionals in some 25 different Centres for PHC performing one or more of the processes distinguished in table A. An interview protocol was designed for each process to be able to 'synthesize the information needs from the utilizing system' rather than just plain asking or looking at existing information systems (Davis' third strategy of information determination [9] was used, in line with the basic assumptions described above).

From a rather classical data analysis of the complete set of information needs, basic requirements, expressed in terms of the information model of the record system in terms of objects, attributes and relations, can be derived.

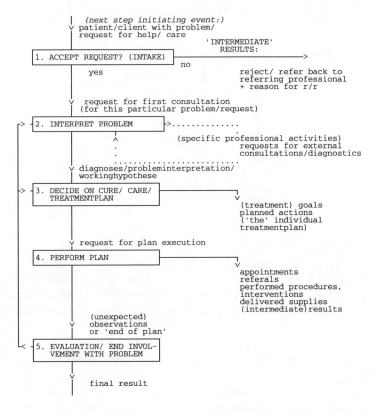

Figure 2. Basic steps in a primary process.

Quality management is not considered to be any different from other management subjects such as production, capacity or resources. On the strategic level one needs to draw up a plan from the mission of the business stating goals and criteria (and values attached) to be met by the primary process and controlled by the managerial control process. The generic structure of this control process is basically a feedback loop, see figure 3.

In this feedback loop a crucial role is played by the first step: the monitoring of 'control parameters'. These are variables which *indicate* the presence of problematic or unexpected behaviour of the primary process: behaviour which is not in accord with to plans, goals or standards. The 'parameters' do in general not *explain* why something is wrong (problematic or unexpected) with the primary process. As a rule there are only a few essential parameters that can be monitored because the monitoring step requires the people executing the primary process to do supplementary data recording, often not needed for the primary work itself. If something exceptional has been monitored then the managerial control process has to find out why: explaining variables (and their monitoring or data collection) are needed.

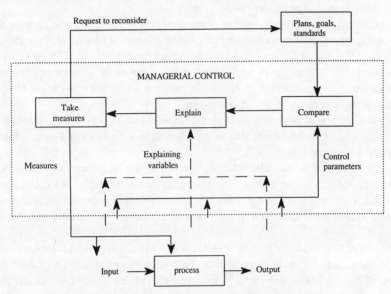

Figure 3. Generic model for managerial control.

This is the second step in the control loop. Third step in the control loop is a choice from two classes of measures. On one hand managerial control will always first try to change the primary process or its inputs. On the other hand if all changes fail to achieve what has to be done the only thing that is left is putting forward requests to the strategic part of the management process to reconsider the plans, goals or standards that have to be controlled. Next step in the loop is of course again the monitoring of the (changed) primary process, comparing the control parameters against (possibly changed) plans and standards.

From interviewing of managers and Delphi methods [10] it has been established that the parameters that are monitored in actual health care organizations come from five categories:
1.   the input of the process, e.g. the number of new requests of a certain type in a given period;
2.   the (efficient) use of the available resources by the process, e.g. the number of performed actions of a certain type versus the needed resources in a given period;
3.   the throughput of the process, e.g. waiting times for patients at different points in the process;
4.   the progress, e.g. results of diagnostic consultations and treatments;
5.   the quality, e.g. the technical quality of performances ('process quality') and the the characteristic features of the outcome of the process ('outcome quality').
Moreover it is considered to be *not feasible* to monitor in an actual health care organization more than about five essentials per process as indicated in table A (and figure 2).

3 Information needed for quality management

In designing an information service for Centres for PHC the authors encountered various unsolved problems concerning quality management. Having modelled the primary business of the centre and the information needed by processes as sketched in the preceding paragraph it is very easy to specify extensive and formal information system requirements for the direct support of processes on the primary level.

But extending these requirements to cover also what is needed by the various activities on the management level concerning quality didn't turn out to be simple. This is caused by the fact that it is not yet clear what the parameters to monitor are if there is an explicit quality plan at the strategic level at all. Because that is maybe the greatest problem: drawing up a quality plan at the strategic level. Such a plan should (in the tradition of Donabedian) contain at least three types of quality related goals:

• goals stating what is needed on *structural* aspects like level of training/education of the workforce, accessibility of the care delivering processes in a financial and geographical sense, availability of equipment etc.

• goals stating what has to be achieved concerning the performance of the *process*, i.e. what business rules including professional guidelines have to be implemented and controlled

• *outcome* oriented goals stating what health or satisfaction improvements for the practice population should be obtained given the initial conditions of the patients and the available resources.

Furthermore this 'total quality plan' should contain a description of the instruments needed to attain those goals. It will be clear that (professional) guidelines are *just* an example. Courses, all kinds of audit, individual instructions, peer review, incentives, sanctions etc. are alternatives frequently encountered in reality. The problem of management is to choose the appropriate mix of quality promoting instruments given the current performance of the care delivering process and its performers and to do so at acceptable cost and effort.

Managers need specific types of information to develop that plan and make those choices. The experience of developing various business information models shows three types of information needed.

Firstly, management has to know the current performance and outcome of the processes for the whole range of health problems encountered in PHC. For example do the GP's in the Centre for PHC deal sufficiently *themselves* with patients with well controlled diabetes mellitus type II, or do they simply refer too often to specialized care (and save time to devote to other agreed work)? The question is of course what is 'sufficiently', and what constitutes good control. To answer this kind of question explicit policies or outcomes of negotiations with financiers are a necessity. This means that the overall health policy (or mission) of the Centre has to be made explicit in terms of patient/problem categories at which the primary process level is aiming its products and services.

Secondly, the manager has to know about the extent to which current performance can be influenced by the introduction of all kinds of instruments e.g. guidelines. Explicit outcome (improved health or satisfaction) related criteria are needed here.

And thirdly, to make the appropriate judgement on what is feasible to introduce as (new) instruments the management has to know about the practical implications of implementing process restructuring instruments like guidelines:

. can they be made acceptable to professionals (can one get consensus, can the instruments be integrated in the daily routines etc.) ?

. are they controllable in the sense that there are control parameters associated with the instruments that can be recorded with acceptable effort by professionals?

These control parameters are not just needed for 'internal' control of the business but are often also needed for accountability reasons in absence of explicit or valid outcome indicators.

4. Conclusions on additional requirements for guidelines

Many requirements on Primary Care Guidelines (PCG's) have been reported. A PCG has to be valid, reliable, clinically relevant and applicable, comprehensive and specific, flexible, clear and understandable, didactic, and attractive [11].

If PHC is going to be more than professionalized art some requirements from a business point of view have to be added. From the experience in the Dutch Centres for PHC the following should be added:

On the primary process level:
• guidelines useful for process quality management enclose at least a part of a primary process which results in a product or service that is distinguished on the business plan level (minimum enclosure is *not* the level of technical procedures of some professional) ;
• guidelines need a simple indicator stating whether it is appropriate to consider applying the guideline right from the start of a process, that is, they need to have an entry criterion;
• guidelines must be explicit about the level of training that is required for optimal use of the guideline.

On the control level:
. guidelines useful to quality management as part of the overall business management cover all the steps of a primary process (as delineated in figure 3), because the 'unit' of control is (in general) not the separate step in the primary process
. guidelines must contain:
-    indicators measuring the preferred outcome
-    valid and feasible (in the sense that an acceptable effort is required) indicators on whether this result of process has been achieved following the guideline

On the strategic level:
. knowledge of the achievable effect of introducing a guideline given the current performance and outcome of the process has to be available for all guidelines to be considered.

Finally, Centres for PHC badly need the results of cost/benefit studies on introducing and controlling the continuous use of guidelines. Every minute that is spent by a professional on using guidelines and reporting to the management must be returned as savings elsewhere in the process (better outcome or less redundant procedures). The Centres need the results of these studies the more because one cannot experiment with the introduction of guidelines in a non-committing 'once only' research fashion, as has been shown in the analysis of Grimshaw and Russell [12].

References

[1]   Grol RPTM. Development of guidelines for general practice care. Br J Gen Pract, 1993, 43, 146-51.

[2]   Thomas S. Guidelines of the Dutch College of General Practitioners (in Dutch: Standaarden van het Nederlands Genootschap). Ned Tijdschr Geneeskd, 1993, 137, 2135-8.

[3]   Lamberts H. In the practice of the General Practitioner: report on the Transition project (in Dutch: In het huis van de huisarts: verslag van het Transitieproject). Lelystad: Meditekst, 1991.

[4]   Foets M, Velden J van der, Bakker DH de. Dutch national survey of General Practice: Survey design. Utrecht: NIVEL, 1992.

[5]   Mulder J, Kroon A de, Duijn J. Prescription policy-making by Pharmacist and General Practitioner in the Netherlands: state of the art and possibilities for improvement? part I&II (in Dutch: Farmacothe-rapie-overleg in Nederland: hoe staat het er voor en hoe kan het beter? deel I&II). Pharmaceutisch Weekblad, 1993, 128, 1236-41 & 1312-6.

[6]   Guidelines for shared care in Centres for PHC, National Union of Centres for PHC (available in Dutch from: Landelijke Vereniging Gezondheidscentra, LVG, Utrecht, the Netherlands): Multiple problems of elderly, 1994; Sleeping problems, Arthrosis, Urinary incontinence of elderly women, Diabetes Mellitus type II, 1993; Stress complaints, Low back pain, 1992; Homecare for the terminal ill, CNSLD in children, Policies on prescription and delivery of drugs, 1991.

[7]   Zanstra PE, Beckers WPA. Computerized assessment with primary care guidelines in the Netherlands. In: Health Telematics for Clinical Guidelines and Protocols. Gordon C and Christensen J P (eds). Amsterdam: IOS Press, (1994).

[8]   Hoopen AJ ten, Nutma J, Boon DA, Boven RF van, Roos V, Vries Robbé PF de. The reference Information Model for Primary Health Care Centres version 1.1 (in Dutch: Het GezondheidsCentrum referentie InformatieModel, versie 1.1). Nijmegen/Utrecht: Vakgroep Medische Informatiekunde, Epide-miologie en Statistiek KU Nijmegen/ Landelijke Vereniging Gezondheidscentra & Stichting Nederlands Instituut Voor onderzoek van de EersteLijnsgezondheidszorg, 1994.

[9]   Davis GB. Strategies for Information Requirements Determination. IBM Systems Journal, 1982, 21(1), 4-30. (reprint) In: Galliers RD (ed). Information analysis: selected readings. Addison-Wesley Publishing Company, 1987.

[10] Geurts-de Haas GE, Oorschot HPF van, Vondel H van. Hospital Information Model (in Dutch: Zieken-huis InformatieModel). Utrecht: NZi, 1984. (NZi; 84.382)

[11] Grol RPTM. Standards of care or standard care? Guidelines in general practice. Scan J Prim Health Care, 1993, 11 (suppl 1), 26-31.

[12] Grimshaw JM, Russell IT. Effect of clinical guidelines on medical practice: a systematic review of rigorous evaluations. Lancet, 1993, 342, 1317-22.

Health Telematics for Clinical Guidelines and Protocols
C. Gordon and J.P. Christensen (Eds.)
IOS Press, 1995

From Guidelines to Decision Support in the Management of Asthma

M. Modell, S. Iliffe,[a] A. Austin and M.S. Leaning[b]

[a] *Health Care, Archway Site, Department of Primary Whittington Hospital, Highgate Hill, London N19 5NF*

[b] *Department of Statistical Science, Clinical Operational Research Unit, University College London, Gower Street, London WC1E 6BT*

Abstract. Asthma is a common chronic disease of the lungs caused by inflammation of the airways affecting 6-7% of the population. Asthma is becoming commoner and there is evidence of under-diagnosis and poor management. Guidelines have been developed aimed at improving quality of care and in reducing social costs of asthma. The paper discusses an approach to implementing guidelines through decision-support systems in primary care, based on methods developed in the AIM GAMES-II project. We also describe a prototype system that has been developed and a programme of clinical evaluation.

1 Introduction and Background

Asthma is a common chronic disease of the lungs caused by inflammation of the airways affecting 6-7% of the population[1]. It is commoner in children than in adults and in a recent study of over 1400 Leicester children 12.7% of boys and 9.2% of girls had been diagnosed as suffering from asthma by the time they were 6 years old[2]. Attacks of asthma may arise spontaneously or be caused by a variety of stimuli including respiratory infections, stress, allergens such as the house dust mite, and air pollution, particularly from vehicle fumes[3]. An affected person will usually cough, wheeze and complain of tightness of the chest and difficulty in breathing. The symptoms are often worse at night and after exercise and may be seasonal. The severity of the disease is very variable; many patients are usually perfectly healthy, wheezing only once or twice a month; others have permanently reduced ability to breathe properly.

A number of studies have shown that asthma has become commoner since the 1970s, especially in children[4]. The rate of admission to hospital has risen steeply over the same period. Though there has been a welcome slight fall in asthma mortality, it is still a third higher than it was in 1977[5,6]. There is also evidence that asthma is under-diagnosed and under-treated and that some deaths are avoidable[7,8]. The social costs are also great, with up to 47% of asthma sufferers missing work or schooling each year because of asthma[9].

The advances in drug treatment in the last 20 years have rendered even severe asthma much more amenable to treatment, though it is not yet possible to reverse the underlying lung pathology. The commonest reason for failure to control asthma effectively is inadequate use of available medication.

1.1 Care of Patients

The majority of asthmatics are looked after entirely within the community. Over 30,000 General Practitioners (GPs) cover the United Kingdom, most of them working in groups of 3 or 4 doctors with other health professionals. These include practice nurses who have a very significant role in the care of people suffering from asthma. It has been estimated that a general practice list of 10,000 registered patients, will include about 60 children and 80 adults with asthma[10]. The importance of asthma has been recognised by the UK Department of Health, and practices that offer systematic care are entitled to extra payments from the Family Health Service Authority (FHSA), the organisation which manages services provided by family practitioners. As with other chronic diseases, the most severely affected patients are looked after by consultants (in respiratory medicine or paediatrics), but even for these patients, care is often shared with the GP.

1.2 Diagnosis

Under-diagnosis probably most commonly occurs in asthmatic children who may present with a nocturnal cough or recurrent respiratory infections rather than with the classical wheeziness or tightness of the chest. On the other hand, wheezing after viral infections in toddlers does not necessarily mean asthma. Certain diseases affecting the chest may mimic asthma leading to diagnostic difficulties. Examples are cystic fibrosis in young children and emphysema in older adults.

1.3 Management

Optimal management of asthmatic patients often includes complex decisions which are difficult in the context of the general practice consultation (which lasts on average 8 minutes). Management plans must be tailored to the individual patient and often depend on how the disease has affected him/her in the past. The plans include instruction, (a) in the use of medications that relieve or prevent symptoms, (b) on the correct use of appropriate drug inhalation devices, (c) in methods of avoiding allergens and (d) on when to seek medical help.

It is now feasible to produce an agreed management algorithm, as consensus guidelines on the management of asthma based on a clearly delineated step-wise approach (step 1. treatment for mild asthma - step 5. treatment for severe asthma) were initially published in 1990[11,12]. The most recent version, incorporating treatment for children was published in 1993[13,14]. These steps are in effect the "gold standard" for asthma management in primary care.

A summary of the stepped approach to the management of chronic asthma in adults is shown in Fig. 1.

A systematic review of the relevant literature concluded that adhering to clinical guidelines may improve the process and outcome of patient care[15]. Decision support systems have also been shown to improve clinicians performance and may produce a significant improvement in patient outcomes[16].

STEP 1 **Occasional use of inhaled bronchodilators** (drugs to immediately relieve symptoms)
STEP 2 **Bronchodilators as needed + regular inhaled anti-inflammatory agents -** **usually steroids** (drugs to prevent symptoms developing)
STEP 3 **Bronchodilators as needed + higher dose inhaled steroids**
STEP 4 **High dose inhaled steroids + regular use of bronchodilators** (rather than episodic use to relieve symptoms)
STEP 5 **Addition of regular oral steroids**

Figure 1. Steps in Asthma Management (adapted from [Guidelines on the
Management of Asthma. *Thorax Supplement* 1993;48:S1-S24])

A computer decision support system may enhance the ability of doctors to diagnose asthma in atypical cases and support management decisions for all primary care workers treating large numbers of people with asthma. It is essential that it compares information obtained at presenting consultations with that acquired during previous encounters between the patient and primary care team. Asthma management is evolving and changing, and decision support systems must be flexible so that they are able to be easily modified to incorporate future changes in therapy.

2 Design Considerations for Decision Support System

The Clinical Operational Research Unit (CORU) at University College London and the UCL Department of Primary Health Care are developing such a system, integrating objective and subjective information about a patient's condition, for testing in the primary care setting. It aims to aid:
a.   diagnosis
b.   assessment of severity of symptoms
c.   development of a therapeutic plan in accordance with the guidelines stepwise approach

d.   monitoring of the patient's progress.

A number of short vignettes were produced by the GP collaborators, covering diagnosis, management and monitoring of patients with asthma of varying degrees of severity. From these, problem-solving algorithms and a set of rules developed.

3   Specification of the Decision Support System: application of the GAMES-II methodology

The prototype system will be an integrated clinical information management and decision support system. The specification for the decision support elements was done using the knowledge modelling methodology developed in the CEC GAMES-II project [19]. The GAMES-II methodology (GM) firstly analyses the generic medical decision making tasks of diagnosis, therapy planning and monitoring, as they apply in a particular domain. The task analysis of patient management in asthma is shown in Figure 2. Following the diagnosis of asthma, treatment planning is concerned with the initial treatment plan and its subsequent adaptation. Monitoring assesses the response to treatment and the general progression of the condition.

GM postulates that a select-and-test model (ST-model) is applicable to all decision-making tasks, regardless of type [20]. An example for asthma diagnosis is shown in Figure 3. Whilst the ST-model is naturally applicable to diagnosis, it appears to be less easily applicable to planning treatment and monitoring.

Assessing Asthma Severity.   Asthma severity is modelled as an abstraction of asthma symptoms and peak expiratory flow rate (PEFR). Each asthma symptom (eg wheeze, shortness of breath and nocturnal cough) is assigned a weight. The symptom weights are summed to produce a total symptom severity score. This is combined with the PEFR measurement in a lookup table to give the asthma severity (Fig. 4). An additional useful variable is the percentage expected PEFR, where the expected value is a function of age, height and sex.

Temporal Change.   The decision algorithm and rules are triggered by the change in asthma severity and by chronic changes in percentage expected PEFR, computed as described above, and compared at successive consultations. A decreasing severity score corresponds to improving asthma, and an increasing score to worsening asthma.

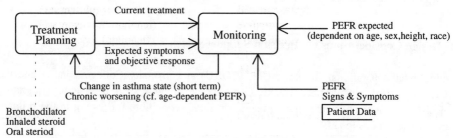

Figure 2. Task model

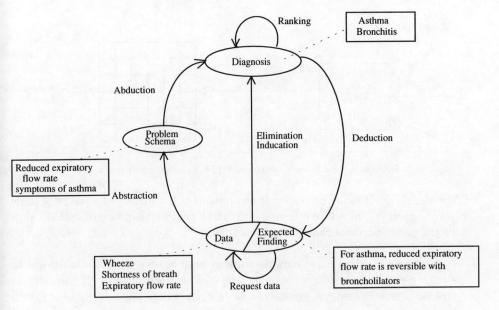

Figure 3. Select and Test Model for Diagnosis [20]

Treatment Planning. Knowledge about treatment planning, embodying the guidelines stepwise approach [13, 14] and additional clinical knowledge, is represented in algorithms and rules. Fig. 5 shows the algorithm for worsening asthma, and Fig. 6 a rule for deciding the need for emergency procedures.

4. CONCLUSIONS

4.1 Implementation and Current Status

A preliminary version of the rules and abstraction functions was implemented, tested and refined in M-KAT II [21], a software package implementing ST-models for diagnosis and treatment planning. M-KAT II was very useful in developing and refining the knowledge-based specification developed here. A clinical prototype system has been developed using Microsoft Visual Basic and the Access relational database server.

4.2 Future Plans

The specification of asthma decision support developed within the GAMES-II project as a test of the GAMES-II methodology has been taken forward by the University College London team in this prototype system. The plans for future development and evaluation are outlined below.

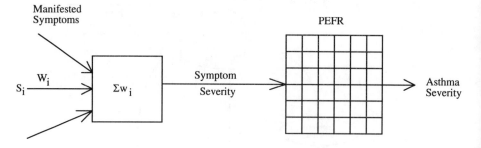

Figure 4. Asthma Severity Assessment (PEFR = peak expiratory flow rate)

The confidence of health professionals and patients in the efficacy of a patient specific decision support system will be enhanced by a careful programme of evaluation[17]. Most of the processes described below will run concurrently.

To be of help to primary care staff, the software must be easy and quick to use and be able to give consistent answers compatible with current expert opinion. It must also be compatible with computer systems likely to be used in practices, and be capable of regular updating. The project team are working with manufacturers of commonly used proprietary GP systems to produce compatible software.

System Validation. The rules and algorithms which form knowledge base of the decision support system will be reviewed and refined by a panel of experts comprising GPs with a specific interest in asthma, practice nurses, respiratory physicians and paediatricians. At the same time, records of approximately 100 consultations with asthma patients will be collected from practices. These will include the actual management decisions made by the GP and practice nurse. The cases will be put through the decision support system and members of the panel of experts will also give their opinion on the appropriate management. The knowledge base will then be refined until it achieves the greatest possible agreement with the expert panel, taking into account actual management decisions made. At the same time, the system will be field tested in a few practices to assess how acceptable it is to potential users. This assessment will be by means of a questionnaire and structured interview. The aim of this process is to improve the way information is presented by the system.

Pilot Evaluation. The objective of this stage is to estimate the likely effect of a decision support system on asthma care. Five pilot practices using the system will be compared with the five control practices. There will be approximately 500 patients in each group. Patients will be interviewed at the start (baseline) and at the end of the pilot phase in both groups. Data will be collected on asthma morbidity and social disruption (using the MacMaster questionnaire[22]), prescribing patterns for asthma in the previous six months, hospital referrals and emergency treatment. Changes in asthma care and outcome for each patient over the pilot phase will be compared between the two groups of practices. It is hoped that this study will provide the information needed to plan a national study of the effectiveness of the system by enabling a calculation of the numbers of practices and patients that will be necessary.

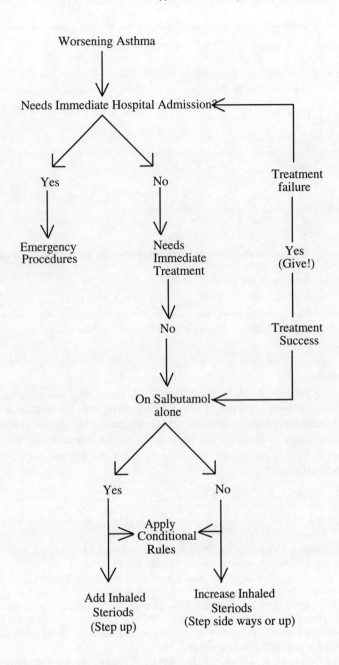

Figure 5. Algorithm for Worsening Asthma

If asthma much worse

and unable to complete a short sentence in one breath

or

silent chest

or

cyanosis present

or

respiratory rate >25/min and not hyperventilating

or

heart rate >110.min and not febrile, not overusing salbutamol and not hyperventilating

Then needs emergency procedures

Figure 6. Rule for Deciding Need for Emergency Procedures

Acknowledgements

This work was conducted as part of the CEC Advanced Informatics in Medicine Programme's GAMES-II project. The Clinical Operational Research Unit is also supported by the UK Department of Health. We are grateful to our colleagues on the GAMES-II project for their helpful collaboration. This paper is based on a chapter in Deliverable 37 of the AIM GAMES-II Project.

References

[1.] Gellert A R, Gellert S L and Iliffe S R (1990) Prevalence and management of asthma in a London inner city general practice. British Journal of General Practice **40**,197-201.

[2.] Luyt D G, Burton P R, Simpson H. Epidemiological study of wheeze, doctor diagnosed asthma, and cough in preschool children in Leicestershire (1993). BMJ 306, 1386-90.

[3.] Breathing in our cities - urban air pollution and respiratory health. Parliamentary office of Science & Technology (1994).

[4.] Peat J K, van den Berg R H, Green W F, et al. Changing prevalence of asthma in Australian children. British Medical Journal **308** 1591-1596 (1994).

[5.] Hyndman S J, Williams D R R, Merrill S L, Lipscombe J M, Palmer C R. Rates of admission to hospital for asthma. British Medical Journal **308** 1599-1600 (1994).

[6.] Ayres J G, Noah N D, Fleming D M. Incidence of episodes of acute asthma and acute bronchitis in general practice 1976-87. British Journal of General Practice **43**,361-365 (1993).

[7.] Carswell E. Thirty deaths from asthma. Archs. Dis. Childh. **60**,25-28 (1985).

[8.] Jones K P, Bain D J G, Middleton M, Mullee M A. Correlates of asthma morbidity in primary care. British Medical Journal **304** 361-4 (1992).

[9.] Clark T J H. The occurence and cost of asthma. Cambridge Medical Publications (1990).

[10.] Barritt P W. General practitioners and asthma Thorax **47** 669-70 (1992).

[11.] British Thoracic Society, Research Unit of the Royal College of Physicians of London, King's Fund Centre, National Asthma Campaign. Guidelines for management of asthma in adults: 1 - chronic persistent asthma. British Medical Journal **301**,651-3 (1990a).

[12.] British Thoracic Society, Research Unit of the Royal College of Physicians of London, King's Fund Centre, National Asthma Campaign. Guidelines for management of asthma in adults: II - acute severe asthma. British Medical Journal **301**, 797-800 (1990b).

[13.] Guidelines on the management of asthma. Thorax **48** S1-S24 (1993).

[14.] Archives of Disease in Childhood Asthma: a follow-up statement from an international paediatric consensus group.**67**,240-8 (1992).

[15.] Grimshaw J M, Russell I T. The effect of clinical guidelines on medical practice, a systematic review of rigorous evaluation. Lancet **342** 1317-1322 (1993).

[16.] Johnston M E, Langton K B, Haynes R B, & Mathieu A. Effects of computer-based clinicial decision support systems on clinician performance and patient outcomes. Ann Intern Med **120**:135-142 (1994).

[17.] Wyatt J, Friedman C, & Spiegelhalter D. Evaluating medical decision-aids. In: Uckun S (ed). State-of-the-art and future directions in AI in Medicine. Elsevier 1994 (in press).

[18.] Juniper E F, Guyatt G H, Epstein R S, et al. Evaluation of impairment of health related quality of life in asthma: development of a questionnaire for use in clinical trials. Thorax **47**;76-83 (1992).

[19.] Lanzola G, Schreiber G & Stefanelli M. Methodological Foundations of Medical KBS Development. Accepted for publication in the Knowledge Acquisition Journal (1994).

[20.] Lanzola G & Stefanelli M. A specialised framework for medical diagnostic knowledge-based systems. Computers and Biomedical Research, 25:351-365 (1992).

[21.] Reference for M-KAT II.

[22.] Evaluation of impairment of health related quality of life in asthma. Thorax 1992;47:76-83.

Secondary and Shared Care

Act Management and Clinical Guidelines

Peter Nicklin[a] and Bruno Frandji[b]

[a] *NHS Information Management Centre, 21 Claremont Place, Newcastle Upon Tyne NE2 4AA, UK*

[b] *SAPHIS, 12 Avenue des Prés, Montigny le Bx. 78180, France*

Abstract Clinical activity has always demanded close co-operation and co-ordination between clinicians and specialities. This applies especially in hospitals and in the future it will apply equally in primary and community care. Co-operation and co-ordination require two things: access to guidelines to control shared, distributed clinical activity, and common access to the patient record. Act management facilitates this by managing the process of care as it passes from one performer to another, enabling each to know at what point in the process (or cycle) they stand, what is expected of them, what is expected of others, and enabling them to access the information that they require. This paper describes act management with reference to guidelines and it is a contribution to the process, presently under way, that is intended to bring the leading examples of act management from the AIM NUCLEUS project and guideline support from the AIM DILEMMA project into close interworking in the same system.

1 Introduction

Clinical activity is characterised by diversity, complexity, and the need for co-ordinated work between a range of disciplines. This has caused great difficulty in the design of clinical information systems. Act management addresses this by providing a broad typology of clinical activities and roles that enable the designers of clinical information systems to tackle these problems in an orderly way. Furthermore, act management has provided a concrete basis for the development of hospital systems that are able to operate with the clinical process. This paper explains the conceptual basis of act management and how it might incorporate guideline support.

Act management was first used in the ESPRIT RICHE project [1] in the development of an open hospital systems architecture. It is now being used in the AIM NUCLEUS project (A2025)[2], the ESPRIT EDITH projects in Italy (E7508) and Ireland (E7509), Hospital 2000 in Portugal (E7510) and the French REFERENCE hospital information system project [3]. Act management concepts have been used in the AIM DILEMMA project (A2005)[4] and the act management model used in RICHE has been incorporated into Version 2 of the UK NHS's Common Basic Specification (CBS).[5]

2 Act Management

2.1 Main components

Act management comprises two main components: *act state* and the *requester-performer relationship*. There are 14 states of act and there are a set of known state transitions. The requester-performer relationship enables a clinical system and its users to manage the clinical process, with each participant knowing their role in relation to others with reference to any specific clinical task. Each of the 14 act states has been assigned to either a requester or a performer.

An *act* is an instance of the provision of care. It is defined and related to other acts through a knowledge base which has *class of act* as its basic component. This knowledge base enables the use of guidelines (or protocols) and it assists the progress of an act though its different states - or through the *act life cycle*. For this reason it is sometimes referred to as *intelligent act management*.

2.2 The Act

An act may be a past activity, it may be in progress or it may be planned for the future. The definition of an act covers any activity provided for the benefit of a patient. An act may generate information about a patient: test results, diagnoses, etc.

Some examples of acts are:
- Consultation
- Visit
- Laboratory test and associated sampling
- X-ray examination
- Collection of vital signs
- Surgical operation and associated anaesthesia
- Drug administration
- Giving meals
- Administering bandages
- Admission to a care unit ...

The atomic level of acts is the *elementary* act and, as might be expected, these can be structured together into *composite* acts which may vary in complexity from a single "thread" of clinical activity to the implementation of a complex guideline supported by a knowledge base (see 2.4 below).

2.3 The Requester-Performer Relationship

Act management makes a distinction between requesters and performers of acts and establishes a relationship between them. In some cases the requester and the performer may be the same person, but the distinction still applies because the requester-performer relationship defines *roles,* not individuals. Requesters and performers co-operate to perform the act at each step of the *act life cycle* (see 2.4 below). This definition is illustrated in Figure 1 using an entity relationship model:

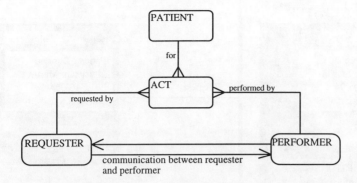

Figure 1 - The Patient, the Act and the Requester-Performer relationship

A requester is any health care professional, physician, nurse, etc. who has the capacity to request the type of act in question. The requester can work in clinical units, in specialist consultancy or in the hospital ward, and has access to the following functions:
- act request
- scheduling of acts (in the case of performer delegation)
- cancelling of scheduled or non scheduled acts
- delaying of acts

A performer is any health care professional who has the capacity to perform the type of act in question. The performer works in care units, in the medical support units, etc. and has access to all functions except act requesting:
- act acceptance, suspension or refusal
- scheduling of acts
- act performance
- act reporting
- cancelling of acts
- delaying of acts

The performer manages the resources required to perform an act, defines the characteristics, the attributes and the environment of the act that he or she performs, throughout its life cycle.

The requester-performer relationship is a key concept, but act management also takes into account any third party concerned with the performance of an act.

Figure 2 (over) illustrates the requester-performer relationship with an example of consultation leading to a request for an abdominal X-RAY, a coloscopy and a gastro-enterologist consultation.

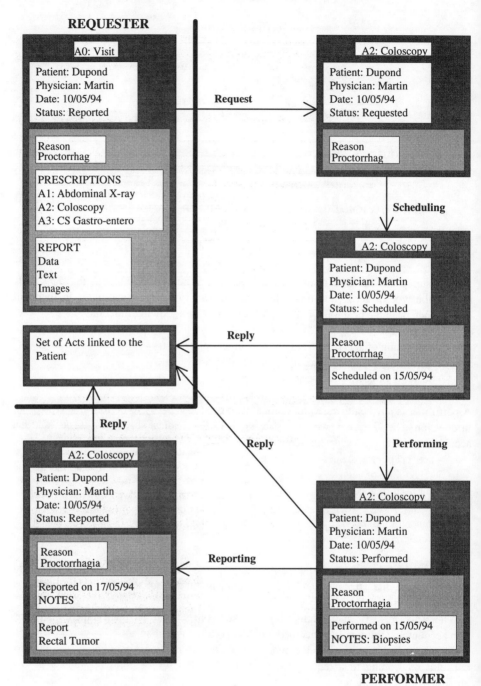

Figure 2 - Requester-Performer Relationship

2.4 The Act Life Cycle

An act has a life cycle. It changes its state according to events. For example:

- the request for an act for a patient, by a *requester* (physician, nurse ...) to a *performer* (specialist, medical support unit, the requester himself, nurse ...),
- the acceptance of the requested act, its suspension or its refusal by the performer (for example for technical reasons),
- the scheduling of acts, usually by the performer, by the requester himself, or by a special third party (e.g. central reservation office),
- the performance of the act by the performer that provides uninterpreted results which are available to the requester,
- validation and interpretation of the results by the performer which are used to produce a report.

This approach allows the act to be represented in a standard way with the assurance of consistency and homogeneity in the system. In particular it makes it possible to apply common functions such as protocol break-down (into sub-protocols or elementary acts), interaction control, scheduling of acts, and act maintenance functions.

Figure 3 shows the state transitions of a number of states, as well as dividing them into the domains of the requester and the performer. The states of cancelled, abandoned and suspended have been omitted from this figure in the interest of presentability.

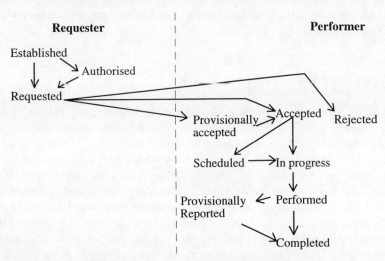

Figure 3 - Act Status, Requester and Performer [Maury 94]

The state transitions shown in Figure 3 were developed as part of the AIM NUCLEUS project [6] and they show a remarkable similarity to the state transitions developed, quite independently, by the AIM DILEMMA project. See Ian Herbert's chapter in this book for these state transitions. This similarity bodes well for the intended convergence of NUCLEUS act management and the DILEMMA project's protocol management.

2.5 Act Management and Knowledge

In act management a distinction is made between the *class of act* (or act type) and the *actual act* performed for the benefit of a patient. The description of the classes of act and their environment corresponds to "knowledge" information as opposed to the operational information attached to patients and to actual acts.

Classes of act provide both a theoretical and a pragmatic description of the provision of health care.

The behaviour of an act throughout its life cycle is described by the attributes of the class of act. The knowledge-base of classes of acts provides, amongst other things:

- hierarchical links between classes of act
- composition links including time constraints
- interaction links including other time constraints
- links with quantified resources
- links with consumable objects including drugs
- links with temporally constrained resources including points of service and point of service sessions

Knowledge is indispensable to the operation of act management and the conceptual design of act management reflects this, enabling a mirror relationship between the operational information (elementary and composite *actual* acts) and knowledge (elementary and composite *classes* of act).

3 Act Management and Guidelines

The transitions of acts between states, the structuring of elementary classes of act into composite classes of act and the division of act states between requesters and performers already constitute a broad form of guidance for clinical activity. Act management forms a framework or skeleton upon which to build knowledge based techniques: semantic and structural links between classes of act, protocol management, clinical guidelines and inference. *Moreover it is a framework that has been designed to utilise knowledge.* As explained above (2.5) act management demands some use of knowledge bases in order to control the relationships between classes of act and these have been incorporated into the NUCLEUS pilot. Indeed NUCLEUS has gone further and has some management of clinical protocols. However much more can be done, especially in the utilisation of advanced guideline support.

Guidelines will increasingly come to be used for the support of shared care where the carers are widely geographically separated. Act management will be a suitable vehicle for this because it will provide the basis upon which widely distributed   carers   can   manage the clinical process using a shared model of the requester-performer relationship and the states of the acts they are concerned with in their work. So for example, an oncology department (*requester*) which is responsible for a cancer patient who is living at home may *request* a district nurse (*performer*) to carry out certain guideline-based procedures, and provide those guidelines to the nurse. The nurse will *accept* the *request* and will then *schedule* her activity. Each separate activity will be an *elementary act* which when *completed* can be *reported* (if necessary) back to the *requester* (oncology department).

4 The Role of the Patient Record

This discussion of act management and clinical guidelines would not be complete without some mention of the patient record. Guidelines are dependent upon good access to operational information. To operate guidelines it is necessary to know about the patient, contra-indications and so on and the results of the whole of a guideline or of some stage of a guideline must be recorded both for future operational purposes and in order to have an adequate clinical audit trail.

Act management is designed to support a *distributed implementation architecture* [7]. This means that a number of *act management servers*, each supporting a department or organisational unit can co-operate with each other in the management of the clinical process and the exchange of clinical information. Act management servers are *objects*. Thus acts provide a patient-centred focal point for the storing of the results of clinical activity such as signs, results and diagnoses. However this does leave this patient information at the point of operation, resulting in a distributed but non-integrated patient record. For this reason the NUCLEUS project has developed the *Patient Reference Dossier* (PRD) to provide a central repository of interrelated references to the patient, HCP, act, result and diagnostic information that is held in different locations.

5 Conclusion

It is intended that the guideline support that is made available by DILEMMA will be made available through an act management/guideline management server (starting with the NUCLEUS act management server). This will be designed to fit within the RICHE open systems architecture, thus enabling it to be exploited by users and system integrators who adopt the RICHE architecture. This process is feasible because DILEMMA and the NUCLEUS and RICHE architectures are based upon the CBS generic healthcare model.

The RICHE architecture is held by a Europe-wide not-for-profit company, Stichting Groupe RICHE, which is jointly owned by a group of hospitals, healthcare systems suppliers and government agencies. These organisations have come together in Stichting Groupe RICHE to promote open health information systems and to find practical means of bringing them about. The advent of an open act management/guidelines server will constitute a useful step in this direction.

References.

[1] B Frandji. Act Management models, ver 4.0, AS-25-0300-002, June 1992. In the RICHE final report in process of printing in series Research Report ESPRIT by Springer-Verlag.

[2] P Nicklin et al. NUCLEUS Conceptual Models, Ver 2, 24 December 1994. Obtainable via NHS IMC.

[3] F de la Porte, Y Harel. Une coopération Hospitaliers/Industriels: le project du S.I.H. REFERENCE. In *Informatique et Santé la revue*, no 15, 4th Trimester 1993, pp 15-18.

[4] SI Herbert, C Gordon, A Jackson-Smale, J-L Renaud-Salis. Protocols for Clinical Care, *Proceedings MIE94,* Lisbon, May 1994, Eds. P Barahona, M Veloso, J Bryant. p33.

[5] NHS, Information Management Centre (IMGE(E)), Common Basic Specifications, Version 2, Generic Model, Birmingham, Oct. 1992.

[6] G Maury. The ALCMs and their Databases, unpublished internal document, AIM NUCLEUS project. Obtainable via NHS .Information Management Centre.

[7] B Frandji, J Schot, M Joubert, I Soady. The RICHE Reference Architecture, in *Medical Informatics* Vol. 19 no 1 Jan-Mar 1994.

Quality Assurance in Clinical Neurophysiology: the ESTEEM project example

M. Veloso[a], S. Vingtoft, M. Carvalho, P. Fawcett, A. Fuglsang-Frederiksen, B. Johnsen, R. Liguori, W. Nix, G. Otte, I. Schofield, M. Sales-Luís,G. Sieben and A. Vila

ªDept. of Neurology, Hospital de Egas Moniz, Lisbon, Portugal

Abstract. This paper describes the current status of the utilisation of clinical practice guidelines (protocols) in the ESTEEM project as one form of the clinical quality assurance procedures considered in the project. The performance of electrodiagnostic studies, in terms of which types of conclusions need to be inferred during the examination plan, is briefly described. The main focus of the paper is a description of an European multicentre clinical audit in the field of Clinical Neurophysiology, using a common data-entry protocol for prospective EMG case collection and assessment with the ultimate objective of building up a multicentre reference database of EMG cases.

1 Introduction (rationale for the use of clinical practice guidelines)

If, on the one hand, we live in an era of abundance of knowledge that physicians can use to improve patient outcomes, the quality of clinical decision making is, on the other, under intense scrutiny. As medical knowledge is expanding, in terms of scientific information and practice findings, so also does contradictory evidence exacerbating the problems of clinical decision making. Resultant variations in clinical practice, together with medical uncertainty and even lack of knowledge, not only contribute to misapplication of resources and available services but in particular may lead to questionable results for patients.

If patients only received appropriate clinical interventions there would be a consequent improvement of the quality and consistency of care and, at the same time, a significant reduction of resource wastage. In other words, there is the need to inform clinicians of the "right thing to do". This is the basis for the emergence of practice guidelines defined as "systematically developed statements to assist practitioner and patient decisions about appropriate health care for specific clinical circumstances" [1]. However, the "right thing" depends on judgements based on personal values, prompting the development of practice guidelines with different aims, such as:

- to reduce the variations between physicians promoting a standard management of medical care

  - to reduce the cost of medical care

  - to reduce the risk of litigation, or

  - to improve the quality of medical care basing it on scientific evidence

In addition, definition of the "right thing" raises important problems requiring a deep reflection as to the implementation of practice guidelines, for example in terms of:

- risk of normalisation of unsound practice
- risk of standardising practice around the average which is not necessarily the best
- risk of preventing progress
- risk of deficient management with individual cases
- risk of "cookbook medicine" preventing individual judgement

In spite of all these problems, clinical practice guidelines are here to stay and it is not surprising that they have the best chance of succeeding if implemented by clinicians, that is by those who are going to use them. The existence of formal methods for developing practice guidelines is relatively recent and derives mainly from the work of David Eddy [2-6]. Steven Woolf [7] classifies the methods for developing practice guidelines as *informal consensus development*, *formal consensus development*, *evidence-based guideline development*, and *explicit guideline development*. Besides describing the differences between these approaches the author also proposes the basic steps for the development of practice guidelines, summarised in table 1.

Clinical guidelines are however only one form of clinical quality procedure receiving a special attention nowadays. Medical audit, defined in the UK NHS White Paper "Working

Table 1 - Methodological issues for guideline development [7]

Introductory Decisions
Selection of topic
Selection of panel members
Clarification of purpose
Assessments of clinical appropriateness
Assessment of clinical benefits and harms
Assessment of scientific evidence
Admissible evidence
Review process
Evaluation of scientific evidence
Assessment of expert opinion
Summary of benefits and harms (i.e. balance sheet)
Determination of appropriateness
Assessment of public policy issues
Resource limitations
Feasibility issues
Guideline document development and evaluation
Drafting of document
Peer review
Pretesting
Recommendations for dissemination, evaluation and updating
Recommendations for research
References

for Patients" [8] as "a systematic critical analysis of the quality of medical care, including the procedures used for diagnosis and treatment, the use of resources, and the resulting outcome for the patient", is another. The present article focuses on the way practice guidelines are being currently used in the ESTEEM project, rather than on the methods for their implementation. A special attention is placed on the ongoing methods of implementing a multicentre reference database containing prospectively collected clinical cases validated by means of a medical audit procedure. A brief discussion focusing on quality assurance aspects and the role practice guidelines may play, in the future, concludes the paper.

2 The ESTEEM project

2.1 Brief overview of ESTEEM

ESTEEM is part of the Advanced Informatics in Medicine (AIM) programme run by Commission of the European Communities. Our goal is to develop a prototype telematics system in Clinical Neurophysiology (Electromyography - EMG) based on two main action lines [9]:

- to build an integration environment - the *EMG-Platform* - capable of managing all information needs in the EMG laboratory from data management to decision making in the context of an European EMG information network, in particular allowing
    - local and remote data storage
    - telecommunication between different EMG laboratories
    - use and test different EMG knowledge based systems
- to implement the following clinical activities
    - clinical standardisation
    - multicentre database with EMG reference cases
    - clinical evaluation

Clinical activities actually represent a major component of the project. They include a standardised specification of the anatomic terms and of the different EMG examination techniques (table 2) complemented by a study on diagnostic criteria of Neuromuscular disorders. A major task consists of collecting real patient cases from the participating EMG centres. A detailed analysis and discussion amongst the clinical partners of examination techniques, planning strategies and diagnostic criteria used in collected cases, which earlier studies [10, 11] revealed to be necessary, are the basis for an audit procedure to seek consensus. This consensus procedure follows the principles of the Delphi Method [12] and is being used to build up a consensus multicentre database.

Table 2 - EMG Examination Techniques

ANATOMIC STRUCTURE	EXAMINATION TECHNIQUE
Nerve segment	Motor nerve studies
	Orthodromic sensory nerve studies
	Antidromic sensory nerve studies
	Mixed nerve studies
Nerve	Blink reflex studies
	F-Wave studies
	H-reflex studies
Neuromuscular Junction	Repetitive stimulation studies
	Single fibre EMG
Muscle	Insertion activity
	Spontaneous activity
	Build-up of recruitment pattern
	Pattern of maximal voluntary contractic
	Motor Unit Potentials
	Turns-amplitude analysis
	Power spectrum analysis
	Single fibre EMG
	Macro EMG

2.2 Examination Strategy in EMG

As illustrated in figure 1, based on a certain number of referral hypotheses together with clinical examination, the clinical neurophysiologist makes an examination plan consisting of set of EMG tests (from the set of examination techniques - table 1) which will make it poss to infer the EMG diagnoses [13].

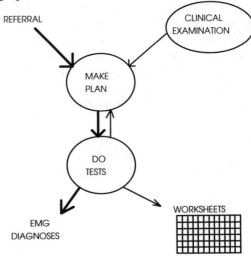

Figure 1 - EMG Examination Plan

Electrodiagnostic data is obtained by applying some examination technique to a certain anatomical structure (figure 2). Results are compared with normal reference values enabling a symbolic interpretation (i.e. normal, mildly increased, moderately increased, severely increased, mildly decreased, moderately decreased, severely decreased, inconclusive, unspecific but abnormal). The use of reference material is a very essential part of the EMG examination. The material is necessary for the objective determination of what is normal and what is abnormal and is based on a set of values defined for each parameter measured on a specific anatomical structure with a given examination technique. Sometimes additional sets of control values exist for different dependencies such as the patient's height, weight, sex, age, segment length and electrode used for the examination. Typically the basis for this reference material is a large amount of data collected from a number of EMG examinations on ordinary "normal" persons, only examined for this purpose.

The rules for the mapping of symbolic values vary considerably among physicians and for examination techniques, examination conditions, etc.. It has been possible, however, within the clinical group of ESTEEM, to obtain consensus on the following general and very simple rules:
- "Normal" is defined as: >= Lower limit AND <= Upper limit
- Lower and Upper limits should reflect the 95% confidence interval
- "Symbols" are mapped according to % deviation or Z-scores.

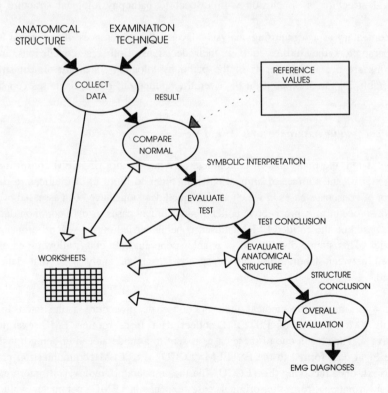

Figure 2 - Test Strategy

PARAMETER NAME	UNIT	VAL	CON	PER	SYMB	NOR	LOW	UP
Conduction velocity	m/s							
Distal latency	ms							
Amplitude (peak to peak)	mV							
Amplitude (p-p) ratio								
Amplitude (negative peak)	mV							
Amplitude (n-p) ratio								
Total area	ms*mV							
Total area ratio								
Total duration	ms							
Total duration ratio								
Negative peak area	ms*mV							
Negative peak area ratio								
Negative peak duration	ms							
Negative peak area dur. ratio								
Number of phases								
Form								

Figure 3 - Motor Nerve Study Parameters

According to the result of the different parameters composing a test (figure 3) it will be possible to state a test conclusion and by evaluating the set of tests applied to the same anatomical structure, a conclusion with respect to pathophysiological structure is also defined.

A complementary aspect requiring analysis concerns the preferences of individual clinicians to the parameters they utilise to base their decisions. Both test conclusions and struct conclusions are declared in terms of the pathophysiological states anatomical structures assume (table 2). Finally, based on the overall examination, EMG diagnoses can be propc [13, 14].

2.3 Clinical Quality Assurance in ESTEEM

As above stated, the main goal of the clinical activities within ESTEEM consortium is to collect a significant number of clinical cases in order to build up a multicentre database consisting of consensus cases in which all contained decisions have been assessed by means of an audit procedure. A prospective collection of clinical cases using a common data entry protocol, based on the entitled EMG data set, is being carried out by seven European EMG laboratories. This standardised protocol enables coherent data entry, allowing cases to be exchanged between laboratories and prospective trials of analysis of that data to be performed.

In figure 4 the multicentre medical audit and consensus procedure is illustrated. In a first phase, all EMG centres of ESTEEM collect data from routine EMG examinations prospectively. Then, each one of these cases is sent to a moderator after being transformed from the local data format to the ESTEEM "ECCO" (ESTEEM communication protocol) format. Next, once receiving this "ECCO" file the "moderator" removes all interpreted and clinical information from the original case except the EMG parameter values, the corresponding symbols and accompanying reference material. Now, such anonymous case is send to all involved EMG experts in ESTEEM who interpret in parallel the case at hand.

Table 3 - Pathophysiologic States [13, 14].

ANATOMIC STRUCTURE	TEST CONCLUSION	STRUCTURE CONCLUSION
Nerve segment	Neuropathic	Neuropathic
	Partial axonal loss	Partial axonal loss
	Complete axonal loss	Complete axonal loss
	Demyelinating / remyelinating	Demyelinating / remyelinating
		Local demyelinating with complete conduction block
		Local demyelinating with partial conduction block
		Local demyelinating with axonal loss
Nerve	Neuropathic	Neuropathic
	Partial axonal loss	Partial axonal loss
	Complete axonal loss	Complete axonal loss
	Demyelinating	Demyelinating
Neuromuscular Junction	Transmission failure	Transmission failure
	Presynaptic failure	Presynaptic failure
	Postsynaptic failure	Postsynaptic failure
Muscle	Neurogenic	Neurogenic
	Myopathic	Myopathic
	Myotonia	Myotonia
	Myotonia with myopathy	Myotonia with myopathy
All anatomic structures	Unspecific	Unspecific
	Impossible	Impossible
	Normal	Normal

Such interpretation includes inferral of relevant test conclusions, structure conclusions and EMG diagnoses. At this stage discussions among the involved experts are not allowed. Once completed, the interpreted case is sent back to the "moderator" who will establish the (dis)agreement level among the local interpretations. If complete agreement is found in the interpretations of all involved experts the case is converted to a final consensus case and placed into the multicentre consensus case database, and the consensus procedure for this case is finalised. If not, the moderator will send back the case to the experts (the minority agreement group) in a second evaluation iteration. Information about the interpretation of the other experts is also enclosed. Evaluators are asked to consider changing their interpretations to be in line with the interpretations given by the majority agreement group. If this is not possible the case will enter a panel discussion and evaluation. The peer review now taking place is still anonymous in the sense that it is not specified from which centre the original case comes from, neither which persons constitute the majority group. If consensus can not be achieved the case is rejected. Otherwise, if consensus is obtained the case is placed into the multicentre consensus case database [15].

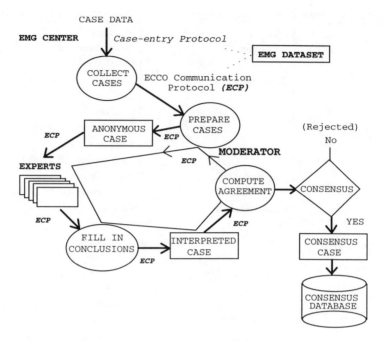

Figure 4 - ESTEEM Medical Audit and Consensus Procedure [15].

3 Conclusion and future developments

How can a clinician assure quality of care in his/her practice? On the one hand, by introducing audit measures for the process of care it is expected that physicians will become more attuned to evaluate critically the quality of their work. In addition, audit constitutes an efficient means to learn and propagate the "best" decisions that should be taken in a given context. This has also been the experience within the ESTEEM project. The ongoing audit procedure has been effective in changing the practice behaviour of involved EMG experts, suggesting that this may be an appropriate vehicle for quality assurance. On the other hand, practice guidelines will help physicians improve their practice from patient data acquisition to patient management and treatment. So far in ESTEEM, practice guidelines have been only used to assure a consistent prospective collection of patient information whose quality is evaluated by means of the above described clinical audit.

However, the resulting multicentre reference data base offers a large potential for future developments [13, 16, 17, 18]. Not only it will be used for a systematised evaluation of EMG knowledge-based systems, one of the major ESTEEM objectives, but also for the implementation and evaluation of practice guidelines in the field. In fact, it provides a sound collection of supporting evidence for the planning, use of tests and decision making during Neurophysiology diagnosis. On the one hand, a clear specification of how conclusions are derived in a given context will allow a more precise definition of the classification criteria for the different conditions. On the other hand, the choice of which test to order (and to perform) should at least partially be based both on the information about how good (valid, reliable, and accurate) the test is in the setting in which the patient was treated and on an explicit estimate of the probability that the patient had the condition for which the test is useful. Carefully selecting the diagnostic tests to use and then using them in a specific order that is conditional on the results of previous tests will not only increase the probability that a correct diagnosis is made, but also that it can be made in a cost-effective manner. In addition, knowledge on how to combine information from multiple tests will lead to better outcomes at the same expenditure level.

References

[1] Institute of Medicine. *Clinical Practice Guidelines. Directions for a New Program*. National Academy Press, M. J. Field and K. N. Lohr, eds., Washington DC 1990.

[2] Eddy DM. *Anatomy of a decision*. JAMA 1990; 263:979-83.

[3] Eddy DM. *Practice policies: where do they come from*. JAMA 1990; 263:1265, 1269, 1272, 1275.

[4] Eddy DM. *Practice policies: guidelines for methods*. JAMA 1990; 263:1839-41.

[5] Eddy DM. *Guidelines for policy statements: the explicit approach*. JAMA 1990; 263:2239, 2240, 2243.

[6] Eddy DM. *Comparing benefits and harms: the balance sheet*. JAMA 1990; 263: 2493, 2498, 2501, 2505.

[7] Woolf SH. *Practice Guidelines, a New Reality in Medicine: II. Methods of Developing Guidelines*. Arch Intern Med 1992; 152: 946-52.

[8] Working for patients. London: HMSO, 1989.

[9] Vingtoft S, Veloso M, Fuglsang-Frederiksen A, Johnsen B et al.. ESTEEM, an AIM project incorporating advanced information processing functions, telematic services and international medical audit into clinical EMG practice, in Barahona P, Veloso M & Bryant J (eds.), Proceedings MIE 94, 1994; 256-260.

[10] Vingtoft S, Fuglsang-Frederiksen A, Ronager J et al, KANDID - an EMG decision support system evaluated in a European multicentre trial, Muscle and Nerve, 1993, 16: 520-529.

[11] Johnsen B, Fuglsang-Frederiksen A, Vingtoft S et al., Differences in the handling of the EMG examination in seven European Laboratories, Electroenceph Clin Neurophysiol, 1994, 93: 155-158.

[12] Kors JA, Sittig AC,van Bemmel JH, The Delphi method to validate diagnostic knowledge in computerised ECG interpretation, Methods of Information in Medicine 1990, 29: 44-50.

[13] Fuglsang-Frederiksen A, Ronager J and Vingtoft S, A knowledge-based EMG expert system for planning and diagnosing (PC-KANDID), Artificial Intelligence in Medicine, 1989, 1: 117-124.

[14] Johnsen B, Fuglsang-Frederiksen A, Vingtoft S et al., A common structure for the representation of data and diagnostic processes within clinical neurophysiology in Barahona P, Veloso M & Bryant J (eds.), Proceedings MIE 94, 1994; 144-150.

[15] Johnsen B, Fuglsang-Frederiksen A, Vingtoft S et al., Observer variation in the interpretation of Budapest 1994: 14.

[16] Schofield I, HINT - High Level Inferencing Tool: an expert system for the interpretation of neurophysiological studies, in Barahona P, Veloso M & Bryant J (eds.), Proceedings MIE 94, 1994; 138-143.

[17] Ziebelin D, Vila A and Rialle V, NeuroMyosis: a diagnostic knowledge-based system for EMG, in Barahona P, Veloso M & Bryant J (eds.), Proceedings MIE 94, 1994; 156-161.

[18] Barahona P, Cruz J, Nascimento S and Veloso M, A causal functional model for anatomo-physiological reasoning, in Barahona P, Veloso M & Bryant J (eds.), Proceedings MIE 94, 1994; 98-103.

The Development of Protocols
to Cover Clinical Care in Cardiology[1]

C.M.B. Duwel and H.A.C.M. Kruijssen

STICARES (Cardiovascular Research Foundation) and Zuiderziekenhuis, P.O.Box 52006,
NL-3007 LA Rotterdam, The Netherlands

Abstract. PROCAS (PRofiles Of CAre System) is one of the AIM projects whose objectives are to improve the quality and efficieny of medical treatment. These will be realised in establishing a methodology for defining and developing what are termed "Profiles of Care". These are sets of options for clinicians which are meant to create acceptable ways of managing patients with similar conditions and which represent good clinical practice. Moreover, a prototype system will be realised by the application of informatics and telematics, to enhance the provision of efficient and effective care in both hospitals and outpatient departments.

Because of the retrospective nature of the ICD-9-CM system for the classification of cardiological patients, a draft for a Prospective Patient Data Model, which involves the assessment of somatic, psychosocial, environmental and demographic axes, is being presented. This multi-axial evaluation allows for the generation of the smallest unit of diagnostic-therapeutic procedures, based on the definition of the patient's health problem; that is: the patient-orientated diagnosis or the appropriate indication.

Introduction

In health care, there is great interest in structuring diagnostic-therapeutic processes. Protocols of care are increasingly mentioned as part of the management of quality of patient care. Problems with the standardisation of patient care include the variability of diagnostic-therapeutic treatment plans and the difficulty of defining (the) patient's health

---

[1] This paper was presented on behalf of the following groups:

The Medical Team of the Department of Cardiology, Zuiderziekenhuis, Rotterdam, The Netherlands: H.X. Krauss MD, PhD, cardiologist; H.A.C.M. Kruijssen MD, cardiologist; W.J. Remme MD, PhD, cardiologist; D.C.A. van Hoogenhuyze MD, cardiologist; C.J. Storm MD cardiologist.

The Committee for Quantitative Information on the Cardiological Profession, of the Dutch Society for Cardiology (QICP): W. Kolsters, MD, PhD, cardiologist (president); C.M.B. Duwel, MD, PhD (vice president); H.A. Schipper, MD, cardiologist; N. van der Putten, PhD, and R.J. van Woersem, MD, cardiologist.

The partners in the European AIM (Advanced Informatics in Medicine) project: PROCAS (Profiles of Care System): P. Di Loreto Ing, Italy; F. Boulay, MD, France; H.A.C.M. Kruijssen, MD, cardiologist, The Netherlands; M. Yates, Belgium; Prof. R.P.P. Jackson, Great Britain.

problem(s). Both are dynamic and change continuously during the diagnostic-therapeutic trajectory.

The PROCAS project

PROCAS (PRofiles Of CAre System) is one of the AIM projects whose objectives are to improve the quality and efficieny of medical treatment [1]. The target of PROCAS is to construct explicit profiles of care, with regard to a group of patients with similar conditions. PROCAS is limited to the medical diagnostic-therapeutic section of care. Nursing and para-medical care, supporting services and hotel services are excluded.

Realisation of PROCAS

The concept of the PROCAS project involves the linking of a specific health problem of a patient (group) with a specific package of care. The latter is a list of optional diagnostic-therapeutic possibilities which play a role in the management of a disease. In the PROCAS project, these lists are called "potential health care plans" and may be connected with a symptom, a sign or a diagnosis.

Current protocols in hospitals

In Rotterdam, several "routines" are part of clinical conditions, having developed in everyday practice. These protocols are explicit standard procedures, with optional diagnostic-therapeutic moments of treatment. At the Department of Cardiology of the Zuiderziekenhuis, the following (episode) protocols of care have been developed: Admission (for Chest Pain), Myocardial Infarction Schedule, Unstable Angina Pectoris or Atypical Chest Pain, Cardioversion, Pacemaker Change, Pacemaker Implantation, Post-Open Heart Surgery; all with a structure comprising a mandatory and an optional scetion. Appendix 1 shows the agreed protocols "Admission" and "Myocarial Infarction Scheme" (version 1.3).

The connection of a symptom, sign or diagnosis with protocols of care

A patient at the Accident and Emergency Ward presenting the symptom "Chest Pain" may receive the diagnosis "(Unstable) Angina Pectoris", which initiates the beginning of the cardiological "Admission Protocol". This includes the immediate execution of the medical procedure of electrocardiography (ECG). If ECG deviations are detected, urgent biochemical laboratory tests are implemented. Positive blood tests (increased enzymes) will lead to execution of the entire admission protocol. Depending on additional characteristics of the chest pain (duration, frequency, severity and associated symptoms) other haematological and biochemical tests, a short intravenous catheter and chest X-ray will be implemented.

The "Myocardial Infarction Scheme" (See Appendix 1) is the first-day component of another protocol, which is activated by the diagnosis of Acute Myocardial Infarction. This is an episode protocol executed over seven days. The first day includes the routines: admission protocol, monitoring heart rate, blood-pressure test, ECG, and haematological and biochemical laboratory tests. Swan-Ganz, intra-arterial or urine catheters, blood gas analyses, echocardiography, heart catheterisation, and haematological and biochemical laboratory tests are optional parts of the protocol and will be implemented according to necessity, i.e. subject to an appropriate indication.

Units of care

Within the Admission protocol, three levels or health problems can be discriminated:
a) Chest Pain
b) Chest Pain with electrocardiogram deviations.
c) Chest Pain, electrocardiogram deviations and increased heart enzymes, i.e., Acute Myocardial Infarction.
If the blood tests are negative, another protocol will be started: the Atypical Chest Pain or the Unstable Angina Pectoris Protocol. The description of some of these health problems may not be found in the classical classificiation system ICD-9-CM [2,3].

Retrospectiveness of the classification system

The objective of the PROCAS project is to register patients in a prospective way. This means that during the diagnostic-therapeutic episode the patient's health problem is described and entered into the system, to generate potential healthcare plans. ICD-9-CM, which should support such classification, is based on retrospectively determined main diagnoses formulated after the patient has left the hospital [2,3]. Moreover, this system is too open-meshed to represent clinical reality.
Diagnostic-therapeutic investigations, medical procedures and drugs are supported by the READ system.

Prospective Patient Data Model

To describe the health problems of patients prospectively, the "problem-orientated diagnosis" and the "(appropriate) indication" are processed into the Prospective Patient Data Model [4]. Both the problem-orientated diagnosis (POD) and the (appropriate) indication (AI) are determined by factors from the somatic, psychosocial, environmental or demographic domains (See Appendix 2). These domains are being studied by the QICP committee of the Dutch Society of Cardiology. Several axes, and within an axis, several factors, may feature in the definition of a POD or an AI.
The development of this model, from the perspective of connecting POD or AI with units of care, is based on the PROCAS concept.

Individual Care

The individual care of a patient will not be threatened: PODs or AIs should adequately describe the individual health problem. The sequence or the profile of PODs or AIs will reflect clinical reality during an episode of care.

Epilogue

PROCAS aims at creating a platform to audit the quality of medical management during an episode of care. This means that a health problem, defined by one or a combination of factors from the Prospective Patient Data Model, will be connected with a unit of care. The consequence of the PROCAS concept is that the PODs and the AIs can define the smallest units of care. These may be part of the computerisation of the order-entry (part of the PROCAS project), the scheduling and logistics of care, or the order-communication system of a clinical information system. A profile of PODs or AIs opens the possibility of creating standard protocols. PODs and AIs offer the cardiologist possibilities in operationalising an audit functionality. This should lead to insight into the qualitative and quantitative performance of cardiological management. Moreover, PODs and AIs present the opportunity to work out the casemix and resource management of patients in a more precise way.

The PODs or AIs as part of the Prospective Patient Data Model require further investigation. They may provide a basis for the realisation of medical audit and the standardisation of care.

References

[1] PROCAS participates in the project line 7: "Regulatory Tools and Quality Assessment" (Mr. John Davies, chairman and Mrs Z. Kolitsi, rapporteur). The AIM project members are: BEAM, DIABCARE, MEMPHIS, ORATEL, PROCAS, QUICHE, SEISMED and TELEGASTRO.

[2] Anonymous. Manual of the international statistical classification of diseases, injuries and causes of death. Volume 1, 9th edition; Geneva: WHO 1977.

[3] Anonymous. International statistical classification of diseases and related health problems. Volume 1, 10th edition; Geneva: WHO 1992.

[4] Duwel CMB, Kruijssen HACM. A draft for a hybrid multi-axial system to classify cardiological patients. 10th International Patient Classification Systems / Europe Working Conference. Budapest, 19-21 October 1994.

Appendix 1

PROTOCOL 'ADMISSION'

This protocol may be carried out:
1) at non-elective admission at the First Aid;
2) at elective admission at the Cardiology Ward;
3) at a diagnostic-therapeutic path at the ward: each determination / investigation is optional.

Haematology:	**Biochemistry:**	**Urine:**
Haemoglobin	Sodium	pH
Haematocrit	Potassium	Protein
Sedimentation rate	Urea	Glucose
Leucocytes	Creatinine	Sediment
Thrombocytes	Alkaline Phosphatase	
Differential count	CPK	
INR (optional)	ALAT	
	ASAT	
	LDH	
	Bilirubin total	
	Bilirubin 1 min (if Bilirubin total	
	has been increased)	
	Total protein	
	Albumin	
	Glucose	

Chest X-Ray AP and Left Lat (optional)
ECG (rest)
Venflon catheter (optional)

CLINICAL GUIDELINES:
- Intravenous Venfloncatheter: if acute treatments are likely.
- Chest X-Ray, which has been carried out in the last 3-6 months will only be repeated if complaints are substantial.

PROTOCOL 'MYOCARDIAL INFARCTION SCHEME' (EMERGENCY TREATMENT)

CLINICAL GUIDELINES:
-     This protocol will be carried out in case of emergency- or non-elective admissions for acute treatment.
-     This routine starts at the CCU.
-     Decision: CCU or Ward based on **ANAMNESIS, ECG (and CPK)**.
-     Patients with thrombolytic treatment during transport in the ambulance should be transferred to the CCU directly.

PROTOCOL ADMISSION (see protocol ADMISSION above)

DAY 1 after 1-2 hrs CCU: (= day of admission)

Protocol monitoring: ECG, rhythm, heart rate, 24 hrs blood pressure
ECG sinus rhythm documenting (optional)
ECG (rest)

1) Swan-Ganz catheter (+pace port) (optional)
2) Intra-arterial catheter (optional)
3) Urine catheter (optional)
4) Blood gas analysis (optional)
5) Echo ± Doppler (optional)
6) Heart Catheterization (optional)
7) Telemetry (optional if transferred to ward)

DAY 1 after 6.00 hrs CCU	**Biochemistry:**
	CPK
	ALAT
	ASAT
	LDH
ECG (rest)	Prothrombin time

DAY 1 after 12.00 hrs CCU:

Haematology:	**Biochemistry:**
Haemoglobin (optional)	Sodium
Haematocrit (optional)	Potassium
	CPK
	ALAT
	ASAT
	LDH
ECG (rest)	Prothrombin time

CLINICAL GUIDELINES:
-     Transfer to the ward: haemodynamically stable patients, no CPK blood enzymes
-     See also CLINICAL GUIDELINES of Day 7.

DAY 2 at 8.00 hr CCU:	**Haematology:**	**Biochemistry:**
	Haemoglobin	Sodium
	Haematocrit	Potassium
	Sedimentation rate	Creatinine
	Leucocytes	CPK
	ALAT	
	ASAT	
	LDH	
	Alkaline Phosphatase	
ECG (rest)	Prothrombin time	

1) Echo ± Doppler (optional)
2) Heart Catheterization (optional)

DAY 2 at 20.00 hr CCU:		**Biochemistry:**
		CPK
		ALAT
		ASAT
		LDH
		Protrombin time

CLINICAL GUIDELINES:
- See Day 7.

DAY 3 at 8.00 hr ward:	**Haematology:**	**Biochemistry:**
or CCU	Sedimentation Rate	Sodium
	Haemoglobin	Potassium
	Haematocrit	Creatinine
	Leucocytes	CPK
		ALAT
		ASAT
		LDH
ECG (rest)		Alkaline Phosphatase

1) Echo ± Doppler (optional)
2) Heart Catheterization (optional)

Patients transferred to the ward (optional)　　　Telemetry

CLINICAL GUIDELINES:
- Haemodynamically stable patients with small infarctions without complications will be transferred to the ward. Patients with large or relapsed infarctions, eldery patients, or patients with complications will stay longer at the CCU.
- See also CLINICAL GUIDELINES of Day 7.

DAY 4 at 8.00 hr WARD or CCU   **Biochemistry:**
                                     CPK
                                     ALAT
                                     ASAT
                                     LDH

Chest X- Ray: Anterior Posterior plus Left Lateral

1) MUGA (optional)
2) Echo ± Doppler (optional)
3) Bicycle ergometry test: age > 65 years (optional)
4) Tc-Sestamibi / Thallium-SPECT (elective)
5) Holter EKG (optional)
6) Heart Catheterization (optional)

CLINICAL GUIDELINES:
-     See Day 7.

DAY 5 at 8.00 hr:

Haematology:	**Biochemistry:**	**Urine:**
Sedimentation rate	Sodium	pH
Haemoglobin	Potasium	Protein
Haematocrit	Creatinine	Glucose
Leucocytes	CPK	Sediment
	ALAT	
	ASAT	
	LDH	
	Alkaline Phosphatase	
	Glucose (fasted)	

ECG (rest)

1) MUGA (optional)
2) Echo ± Doppler (optional)
3) Bicycle ergometry test: age > 65 years (optional)
4) Tc-Sestamibi / Thallium-SPECT (optional)
5) Holter EKG (optional)
6) Heart Catheterization (optional)

CLINICAL GUIDELINES:
-     See Day 7.

DAY 6 at 8.00 hr:	**Haematology:**	**Biochemistry:**
	Sedimentation rate	Sodium
	Haemoglobin	Potassium
	Haematocrit	Creatinine
		CPK
		ALAT
		ASAT
		LDH
		Alkaline Phosphatase

ECG (exercise-) at an age of < 65 years

1) MUGA (optional)
2) Echo ± Doppler (optional)
3) Bicycle ergometry test: age > 65 years (optional)
4) Tc-Sestamibi / Thallium-SPECT (optional)
5) Holter EKG (optional)
6) Heart Catheterization (optional)

CLINICAL GUIDELINES:
- See Day 7.

DAY 7: DISCHARGE

CLINICAL GUIDELINES:
- A MUGA will be executed for the evaluation of ischaemia, complications, ejction fraction;
- An echocardiography will be executed for the evaluation of ischaemia, complications, ejection fraction;
- A bicycle ergometry test will be executed for the evaluation of exercise tolerance, left ventricular function;
- A Tc-Sestamibi /Thallium-SPECT will be executed after a positive stress ECG, for the evaluation of ischaemia or anginal pain;
- A Holter ECG will be executed for the evaluation of arhythmia and AMI.

- Patients with large or relapsed infarctions, the elderly patients, or paients with complications have an average stay of 12 days.

Appendix 2

THE PROSPECTIVE PATIENT DATA MODEL

FACTORS DETERMINING "THE PROBLEM-ORIENTATED DIAGNOSIS" AND "THE APPROPRIATE INDICATION"

The somatic axis consists of the following factors:
1)   the current complaint, rated on an ordinal or continuous scale;
2)   the reason for referral (as diagnosed by the specialist);
3)   the current symptom, rated on an ordinal or continuous scale;
4)   the (current and/or former) primary diagnosis, rated on an ordinal or continuous scale;
5)   the secondary diagnosis, rated on an ordinal or continuous scale;
6)   the most important (deviant) finding of examination, rated on an ordinal or continuous scale;
7)   the interpretation of the result of examination;
8)   the (most important) therapeutic intervention or surgery;
9)   the complication;
10) the current therapy;
11) the (family) risk factors.

The other axes are:
12) the psychosocial domain (problems in/with the family, problems in connection with the social environment, vitality, profession, marital status);
13) the environmental domain (observation, limited access to medical services, research purposes);
14) the demographic domain (age);
15) the functional status (which rates the health status of a patient)].

Protocol-Directed Shared Care in Cardiology

David Pitty, Philip Reeves, Anthony Rickards

Information Directorate, Royal Brompton Hospital, Sydney Street, London SW3 6NP

Abstract. In the new market-oriented UK National Health Service, hospitals succeed or fail on the quality of service they provide to their customers. It is therefore important that institutions like the Royal Brompton Hospital can meet the information and communication needs of General Practitioners and hospitals who use their services so that co-ordination between healthcare professionals involved in the co-operative care of individual patients can be ensured. One method of improving the relationship between healthcare professionals is by the use of consensus-based clinical protocols which define 'best practice' co-operative care for a particular condition. The Royal Brompton Hospital has been a clinical partner in the AIM project DILEMMA which has been examining technology and methodologies for applying clinical protocols supported by telematics to general practice and shared care. A detailed requirements analysis has been carried out to look at the problems of shared care in cardiology and this has resulted in a demonstration system being developed to show how protocol-directed shared care and its supporting technology could be implemented to solve real clinical problems. Conclusions have been drawn that concern the use of protocols and information technology generally in routine clinical care.

1 Introduction

In a relatively short time the practice of cardiology has changed out of all recognition. Just 30 years ago pacemaker implants, coronary surgery and a whole range of minimally invasive interventions were unavailable so the vast majority of patients were managed within a narrow range of therapeutic options which restricted the scope of medical decision making. Tody's 50 year old medical practitioners were trained at a time when modern therapeutic cardiology did not exist. The communication and training overhead required to disseminate new information as close to the point of care as possible is enormous and the problem gets geometrically worse as new treatment methods are introduced. It may not be possible for future generations of healthcare professionals both to deliver care and keep abreast of all therapeutic options available to them.

Continuity, quality and cost effectiveness of care across primary, secondary and specialist centres is therefore difficult due to lack of consensus and common understanding between healthcare professionals, and poor dissemination of knowledge. In cardiology in particular, the rapid expansion of options combined with a culture that does not encourage continued medical training has disadvantaged some sectors of the population. These problems arise from poor communication between the parties involved and a lack of structure for exchange of information. The use of clinical protocols with supporting technology may help to improve this situation.

Under the umbrella of the European Union AIM (Advanced Informatics in Medicine) research programme, the DILEMMA project has been developing generic models and tools to support the design and development of clinical decision support systems, with the emphasis on support for protocol-directed shared care. This work is based on knowledge-based decision support technology that was developed and applied to Oncology during the LEMMA project [1]. The Royal Brompton Hospital (RBH) has undertaken Workpackage 8 of DILEMMA to assist the development of generic technology by evaluating and extending the new models and tools when applying them to a scenario in cardiology [2,3]. The deliverables of this work have been a detailed analysis of shared care in cardiology concentrating on the problems associated with shared care management of patients with coronary artery disease, and a demonstrator system known as PARSEC which shows how protocol-directed shared care may be utilised in this domain to solve genuine clinical problems.

2 Method

The difficulties we are facing in this work are widely accepted; neither expert systems nor decision support systems developed for healthcare have been well received by clinical users and hence there are few such systems in clinical use [4]. Various reasons for this have been proposed such as dependency on 'computer artefacts' and ignorance of organisational constraints [5]. Our initial analysis also highlighted clinicians' fears of 'protocols' or 'guidelines' whether these terms were used in the context of a convenient method for encapsulating knowledge or in the context of protocol-directed care. Although protocol-directed care is prevalent in oncology, there are no widely accepted explicit guidelines for the management of coronary artery disease (CAD) across the referral chain.

Not surprisingly then, when introducing inferencing systems into clinical practice for routine use away from the direct control of the product champion, there is immediate resistance simply because of the threatening terminology used to describe the system. This problem has undoubtedly contributed to some earlier failures and so led us to follow a conceptually different approach. We broadened our requirements analysis to a more general software engineering approach looking at the whole process of clinical management of CAD patients across the referral chain. This allowed us to gain a much more accurate view of the requirements for shared care clinical systems generally, rather than for decision support systems or systems to support protocol-directed care alone. During this process we have attempted to highlight the major problem areas associated with the shared care of patients, and this has been augmented by studying hospital medical records and recording information flow.

Object oriented analysis techniques were used to model the problem domain and this was followed by an object oriented design and the use of an object oriented programming language for the implementation of PARSEC.

3. Problem Identification

When a patient presents with cardiovascular disease requiring treatment there are, in the UK at least, typically three groups of healthcare professionals involved in management of the patient. The primary care physician (General Practitioner, GP) has the responsibility to detect the probability of a serious condition either by clinical means alone or by arranging limited and appropriate investigations. A decision may then be made to refer the patient for more specialised opinion or investigations in a local District General Hospital. Here, most of the GP's investigations will be unnecessarily repeated, wasting time and money, before further tests are made. A decision is made on whether to refer to a specialist centre. Again, communication tends to be poor and many if not all investigations will be repeated before a therapeutic decision is taken and implemented. After therapy the patient will probably attend follow up clinics at the specialist centre which may be many miles from the patient's home, even though it may be technically possible to perform the examination locally. This process is obviously wasteful of patient time and is expensive in terms of medical time and cost of investigations.

When we asked clinicians about ways of improving shared care they were all agreed that the most important requirement was to improve the availability of all clinical information relating to the patient such as medical history, current treatments and so on. In particular they wanted to have access to the management plans of other healthcare professionals, access to test results, and on-line reference information. On further analysis it was found that supporting reasoning for decisions made at other sites was required along with the management plan and shared patient record, interpretation was required along with results, and context sensitive reference information was required due to the vast quantity of medical literature available. It also became apparent that in a rapidly expanding medical discipline the communication of knowledge relating to the selection of the best therapeutic option is extremely difficult, and this is made worse by the lack of consensus in terminology and interpretation which is compounded in rapidly advancing disciplines.

These results were supported by an analysis of past cases [6] where many problems relating to shared care were identified. Patient records were selected randomly from the medical records store at the Royal Brompton Hospital. On detailed examination, every case exhibited situations where care could have been improved, or the process made easier by the enhanced availability or presentation of information. For example:

a. A GP refers patients to his local hospital for Exercise Tolerance Tests. The hospital reports the results back to the GP as a number on a scale of 1 to 5. The GP interprets this scale in the opposite order to the hospital.

b. A district general hospital transfers a patient to RBH for further investigation. With the patient they send the following documentation: referral letter, photocopy of notes relating to the current episode, transfer letter from the ward sister. There is considerable duplication between these documents, and some of the details in the ward sisters letter are wrong (they are a recapitulation of an error made in the notes which was subsequently corrected).

c. A patient is intolerant of aspirin because of an ulcer. This is recorded in near-illegible handwriting in the notes. It is not on the front cover of the notes (as it should be) or in any prominent place. The notes show that doctors were considering treating with aspirin if the patient was unable to have immediate surgery. They seemed to be unaware of the intolerance which was buried away in another part of the notes.

d. A patient suffered an acute myocardial infarction and was admitted to his local hospital. Two weeks later he transferred to RBH because of continuing unstable angina. The notes show that the admitting doctor did not know whether Streptokinase (or other thrombolytic therapy) had been given post-infarct. This meant that if the patient had suffered another infarct then possibly vital thrombolytic therapy could not have been given due to lack of information.

e. A doctor receives a discharge letter concerning a patient which says "Angiography showed this patient to have multi-vessel disease, we have opted for medical management". The doctor knows that a patient with multi-vessel disease would normally require bypass surgery and wonders why this option has not been chosen. The discharge letter does not explain the reasons for choosing a different therapy option.

4 Potential Solutions

From the problems identified, it is clear that some method of co-ordinating the various roles of healthcare professionals is required. As a basic building block, a patient record shared between all healthcare providers would help to prevent repeated investigations and could solve the problems of data duplication and inconsistency. There is no fundamental reason why the patient could not carry details of all observations and treatments throughout the period of care. In some cultures, usually where resources are limited, this is effectively carried out by the patient carrying their own medical records but this makes audit, research and prospective management of workload difficult. In an advanced medical system where both patient and professionals need access to medical data the only realistic way to share information is by using telematics links between the healthcare providers to supply a common medical record.

Once a shared medical record is available the problems of interpretation of clinical terms can be approached. This can be achieved by sharing a common knowledge base containing the terms, their definitions, and relationships between terms so that the interpretation of data is defined as well as the result itself. Terms such as 'Exercise Tolerance Test Result = 1' would thus be understood in the same way by specialist and general physician alike. Ideally, entry of data to the shared patient record would be constrained to the terminology held in the knowledge base so that every data item in the patient record is well defined. However, in practice this is difficult to achieve because of the vast size of the medical domain and lack of consensus between healthcare professionals.

Use of decision support technology that can access the knowledge base and patient record can then be applied to solve some further problems. To augment the shared patient record, context sensitive reference information can be supplied based on the individual patient being treated, along with medical knowledge usually only available to specialists. Decision support watchdogs can monitor prescribing to alert clinicians to drug intolerance, interactions and other contraindications, and explanations for clinical decisions made at other sites can be provided.

With these building blocks in place it is possible to support protocol-directed care and reap even greater benefits. A protocol or guideline agreed between the various players in the healthcare process acts as a structure for the process of co-operatively caring for individual patients. For example, the protocol defines what tests should be performed before referral given a particular condition, and the decision support system can be used to check that patients are not referred without the agreed set of tests being done. Likewise once the protocol has defined which tests are appropriate, unnecessary tests and investigations can be prevented. The specialist gains from a consistent referral pattern and can schedule follow up clinics to be carried out closer to the patient's home. Thus savings in patient time, medical time, and resources can be realised.

New protocols can be developed jointly by specialist and non-specialist physicians according to a defined 'consensus' process, and the new knowledge relating to 'best practice' can then be disseminated to other practitioners. Suggestions for therapeutic options available can be presented and in the case of new treatments or evidence based protocols the supporting knowledge or reference source is also available, so non-specialists always have the option of using a modern treatment or investigation when appropriate.

As a clinical protocol logically determines the sequence of investigations, when decision points are reached and what treatments are available, it is then possible to use this information to implement resource management in real time, that is scheduling of human resources such as surgeons, nurses etc. and non-human resources such as theatre sessions, ultrasound scanners and so on. So by specifying a protocol the day to day operational functions of a healthcare site can be managed.

5 The PARSEC Demonstrator

5.1 Design Principles

It is evident that protocol-directed shared care will improve the continuity, quality and cost effectiveness of care and we have looked at some of the technologies required to support it. However, when considering using computer systems for the practical implementation of protocol-directed shared care, the more generalised requirements for introducing information systems into routine clinical care must be given priority [7]. The design concept for PARSEC (PAtient Records for SharEd Care) is therefore to build a clinically useful tool that incorporates protocol-directed shared care and its supporting technologies, based on three main requirements from our requirements analysis [6]:

- To capture patient information (at the point of generation).
- To use that information to support patient management.
- To make that information available, in the appropriate way, to other healthcare workers.

The system therefore incorporates the following functionality to support these requirements:

- Intelligent support for data entry and patient record browsing.
- Decision support in diagnosis, treatment selection, protocol management and care planning.
- Support for service requisition and provision via messaging functions.

The architecture of PARSEC is explained in the following sections.

5.2 The Shared Patient Record

Our requirements analysis highlighted the importance of information availability and how seemingly trivial data can assume great significance. Some approaches propose models of information sharing where the information originator decides what to send to others but these paradigms cannot satisfactorily cope with the context-sensitive nature of information, with the detailed and varied information needs of multiple carers nor with changes in technology, clinical practice and healthcare delivery. Nor can such a system deliver the potential benefits of an integrated care plan as proposed in [8]. Our approach has been to address these needs by ensuring that all carers have access to the whole of the computerised record at all times, although their views of that record may be different.

We provide user interface components such as care plans and forms which access the patient record via a system component called the Database Manager (see Figure 1). The interface components and the Database Manager share a common view and interpretation of the patient record based on domain and patient record models. In the current implementation of the demonstrator all records are held on a stand-alone PC in DOS files. In future, the patient record could be distributed and composed of information held on different types of systems without changing the system architecture or component interfaces. This is possible because of the single point of access to the patient record through the Database Manager. The Database Manager takes responsibility for retrieving data from wherever it is stored and providing a 'virtual' patient record [9] to other system components. Many possible models for the distribution of information can thus be supported without the need for 'send / receive' messaging for patient information.

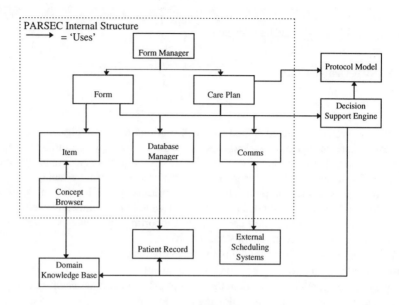

Figure 1 - PARSEC Block Diagram

Messaging functions are still required, however, for the requesting and co-ordination of care services, such as booking catheter labs, nurses etc., and these are provided by the Comms (communications) component. These services can be driven automatically from a defined protocol. Under this scheme users no longer need to consciously send information to others - their sole concern is for the accurate and complete recording of their own healthcare activities and for carrying out those activities.

5.3 Human Computer Interface

The development of computer systems for capturing clinical data is often motivated by the perceived weaknesses of paper notes, for example single-user access, illegibility, susceptibility to loss, difficulties of transfer, poor presentation of information, no interrogation facilities etc. But such systems often overlook the positive attributes of paper notes such as flexibility, speed, and familiarity [10,11]. In the design of PARSEC we have attempted to retain the positive features and overcome the shortcomings by simulating the existing paper medical records for data capture as well as allowing the data to be browsed and summarised in ways that the paper record cannot support.

A set of patient notes on paper generally consists of a largely unstructured collection of forms organised only by their physical order, which may or may not be logical. In PARSEC, a patient record consists of a structured set of forms, managed by the Form Manager component, from which information can be selected, ordered and displayed in a variety of ways. Each Form is a piece of 'smart A4 paper' which acts as a repository for many different types of data. The data entered on the forms is stored independently of the form definitions so the user is not restricted to a form-based view of the record.

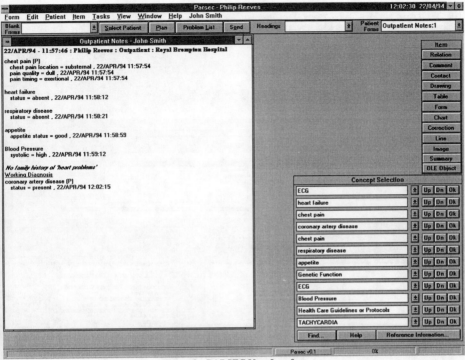

Figure 2 - PARSEC User Interface

Figure 2 shows the user interface of PARSEC with the smart A4 on the left hand side emulating an Outpatient Note.

5.4 Data Items

In PARSEC, Forms contain Items such as Comment, Contact, Drawing, Table etc. which are added to a form by clicking the appropriate button (see Figure 2). Clinical Concepts, such as chest pain, are a type of item but are expressed by selecting them from the Concept Selection window which is an interface to the task-oriented knowledge base browser. The browser provides twelve entry points to the knowledge base as shown at the bottom right of the PARSEC screen in Figure 2. Each concept has a set of attributes such as status (present, absent), duration and location which are derived dynamically from the domain knowledge base. The values of the attributes are set by the user along with temporal information and the concept is then written on the form. Figure 3 shows the attributes for chest pain and the values that can be selected for chest pain location.

PARSEC supports healthcare professionals in their use of drawings to illustrate examinations or investigation findings by supplying a range of predefined drawing templates such as a torso, heart etc., which can be selected, edited with drawing tools and then added to the form. New templates may be added using a system administration function. PARSEC forms can also contain condensed versions of images such as x-rays and CT scans which can be viewed full-size by right-clicking with the mouse on the image. Figure 4 shows an echocardiogram as part of an Echo Report form (reproduction is poor without colour). Using the Microsoft Windows OLE (Object Linking and Embedding) mechanism, a PARSEC form can contain data generated or managed by other Windows

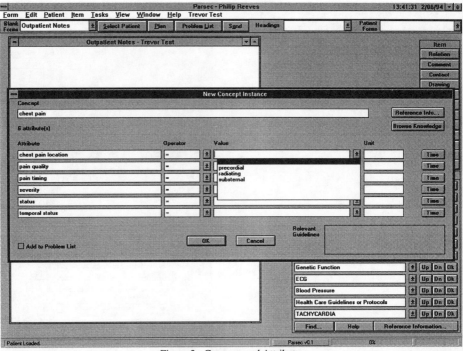

Figure 3 - Concepts and Attributes

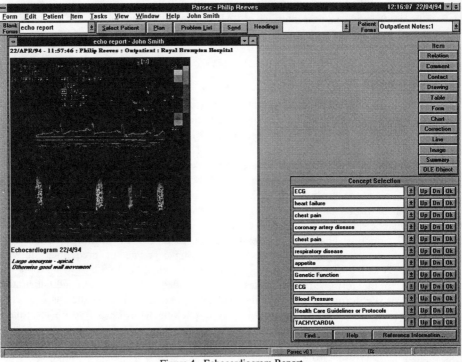

Figure 4 - Echocardiogram Report

applications which allows PARSEC forms to contain multimedia information such as ECGs, angiograms and voice annotated x-rays.

5.5 Decision Support and Protocol-directed Care

Decision support facilities for diagnosis, protocol selection, care planning and drug alerts are provided in PARSEC by way of a Decision Support Engine (see Figure 1) developed within the DILEMMA project consortium. The decision support engine, also known as the Toolset, includes explanations of its reasoning.

For the selection and management of protocols PARSEC has a module dedicated to the graphical representation of the protocol in the form of a Care Plan. The module is compliant with the Generic Protocol Model (GPM) [12] developed within the consortium to provide a structure for representing protocols in any medical specialty, and this module is also integrated with the Protocol Task Manager (PTM) [13,14] component of the Toolset. The user can view the care plan over selected time scales and by selecting the appropriate clinical procedure, have access to all the reasoning which led to the procedure being in its current state, that is the indications which apply to the patient. Reference and background knowledge about the procedure, for example side-effects, outcome evidence etc., is also available. The Care Plan is shown in Figure 5.

As an alternative to following recommendations based on a protocol, the physician may manually amend the care plan and PARSEC will check this amendment for validity against the protocol - this is known as critiquing. The care planning function also has integrated support for requesting and reporting service provision using the Comms component so that

Parsec Patient Plan - John Smith								12:09:47 22/04/94	
Plan Protocol Patient Help John Smith Zoom In! Zoom Out! Recommendations!									
Days	19/APR/94	21/APR/94	23/APR/94	25/APR/94	27/APR/94	29/APR/94	01/MAY/94	03/MAY/94	
Clinical Events						chest pain coronary artery disease			
Relevant									
Established			IHD1 ANBC						
Discarded									
Requested									
Accepted									
Scheduled			Anti hy Weigh Referr ECG			Follow up appointment			
Started									
Cancelled									
Rejected									
Suspended									
Performed									
Abandoned									
Reported			Blood						
Action Validated						Parsec v0.1		0%	

Figure 5 - PARSEC Care Plan

when a test is scheduled, the system can communicate directly with a booking system to see if the relevant facilities and staff are available.

5.6 Summarising Data

One method of adding value to information is by interpretation, for example by creating a summary of various types of information to meet a clinical need. Examination of patient notes shows that clinicians often summarise the patient's history and progress at the start of each consultation to ensure that all relevant clinical information is noted. In addition clinicians find it easier to present to a patient on a ward round from their own notes rather than from someone else's. Summaries are also required for requesting services and reporting on service availability. By the use of the shared patient record, summaries can be created by any clinician, technician, manager, service requester or service provider.

PARSEC forms can be used for generating summaries as well as for data entry by use of Summary Items which specify a set of information to retrieve from the record. When the form containing the item is viewed the summary item is replaced with the specified information, for example the current problem list. PARSEC allows concepts to be categorised under Headings such as Family History thus providing a mechanism that allows information from different parts of the concept hierarchy to be related. These headings can also be referenced by Summary Items. Information can also be summarised by means of Chart Items such as graphs, pie charts and other diagrams. PARSEC can also produce tabular summaries in the form of Table Items.

6 Conclusions

6.1 Use of Protocols

One of the most important conclusions of our work is that there is a problem with co-ordination in shared care. The evidence suggests that primary care physicians do not know enough about what is happening to their patients because of poor communication links with other sites. The problem is compounded because, for example, when a patient attends a secondary or tertiary centre it can often be a daunting experience and consequently communication between the specialist physician and the patient may be unsatisfactory. This makes life difficult for the primary care physician who is expected to be the patient's 'champion' in the healthcare system because they are the most accessible physician for the patient, they see the patient most often, and they receive the majority of the patient's enquiries. However, it seems that primary care physicians are not getting the information they need and so it follows that anything that assists GPs by giving them greater access to information will improve the quality of patient care. Similarly, if specialists can be confident of a consistent level of investigation prior to referral they could save time and money by eliminating costly reinvestigation. A guideline or protocol provides a structure for sharing information by defining the interfaces between healthcare professionals, i.e. when to refer and what should have been done and checked prior to referral, and the protocol also defines the data set that should be shared.

Although the concept of protocol-directed care may appear threatening to medical practitioners, it is nothing more than moving the skills and disciplines of clinical research into routine medical care. Indeed the prospects for medical research to take advantage of such systems is enormous. It is important that the protocols themselves are arrived at through consensus views of primary, secondary and specialist physicians so that the co-ordination of care works in practice. Deviations from the protocol can be tracked and fed back to the protocol definition process, creating modified but validated protocols or creating new protocols. Outcome analysis can also be applied to cases that have followed particular protocols and the results can be fed back to the protocol definition process. This technology also has clear potential for supporting multi-centre clinical trials, since these usually involve protocols.

6.2 Supporting Protocol-Directed Shared Care

We have shown that continuity, quality and cost effectiveness of care could be improved by agreeing 'best practice' between shared care sites, agreeing on a data set required to support the defined best practice, and then distributing that data set between all parties involved in the shared care of a patient. It is possible that traditional telephone and fax methods could be used to support this process and our research suggests that communication such as this will improve the quality of patient care. However, in practice this approach is unlikely to work due to the quantity and diversity of techniques used to capture data about a patient (ECG, x-ray, ultrasound, text, free hand drawing, etc.), and the potential number of participants in the shared care process. But the biggest hurdle to implementing protocol based care into routine clinical practice is the organisational changes required to support a different paradigm of clinical care. Therefore a number of supporting technologies are required before the real benefits of protocol-directed shared care can be realised in day to day clinical practice:

- A shared patient record that is available to all healthcare professionals with a user interface customised to support their particular role in the healthcare process.
- A common knowledge base of terminology with definitions of the interpretation of each clinical term to ensure semantic consistency in the shared patient record.
- A generic model for the structure of protocols that is independent of any particular medical domain.
- A decision support engine to support protocol management and assist in the provision of context sensitive information.

6.3 Building Clinically Useful Systems

Telematics naturally lends itself as a vehicle for implementing the required technology, but our research has shown that the use of this technology introduces a further set of problems relating to the application and acceptance of the technology itself in routine clinical care. These problems can be minimised by:

- Ensuring that a broad requirements analysis is undertaken that examines the complete clinical scenario rather than assuming at the outset that some particular technology or method (such as decision support, protocol-directed care) will be used.
- Using traditional software engineering techniques (such as OOA\D) for requirements analysis and design and only target advanced technology at relevant design modules.
- Using high quality user validated user interfaces. Even the most perfectly engineered advanced technologies will not be accepted into routine clinical use if the overall system is not easy to use.

6.4 Further Work

Based on detailed work with clinicians, analysis of medical records, and study of data flows between healthcare sites, we have concluded that protocol-directed shared care will solve significant problems with shared care in cardiology. We have also demonstrated where information technology is appropriate and where care should be taken with such technology. However, our conclusions have yet to be verified by practical implementation.

The Royal Brompton Hospital has recognised the potential for protocol-directed shared care and so we are continuing this work on a practical level by working with several groups of General Practitioners to define shared care protocols for the management of angina and asthma. In addition we are seeking to continue this work on a more standardised and European level under the Fourth Framework programme of the European Union, using mature technologies assembled from the results of the current Third Framework projects.

References

[1] Renaud-Salis J L, Taylor P. The Bordeaux Oncology Support System: Program Documentation. Deliverable of the LEMMA project, 1990.
[2] AIM Project A2005. DILEMMA Technical Annex, 1994.
[3] Reeves P I, Carniel B, Gibbs S. Decision Support in Cardiology Shared Care: The DILEMMA Project. Proceedings of Computers in Cardiology, 1993.
[4] Cramp D, Goodyear O M. Report on a European Survey. Expert Systems in Medicine, Healthcare Informatics Foundation 1989.
[5] Heathfield H A, Wyatt J. Philosophies for the design and development of clinical decision support systems. Meth Inform Med, 32:1-8, 1993.
[6] Reeves P I, Carniel B, Rickards A F. Requirements for Shared Care Decision Support in Cardiology. Internal Deliverable of the DILEMMA Project, 1993.
[7] Pitty D L, Reeves P I. Developing Decision Support Systems: A Change in Emphasis. Proceedings of Medical Informatics in Europe, 1994.
[8] Rigby M J, Roberts R, Williams J G. Objectives and Prerequisites to Success for Integrated Patient Records. Proceedings of Medical Informatics in Europe, 1994.
[9] Wallace S. The Computerized Patient Record. BYTE, May 1994.
[10] Tange H J. The Paper-Based Patient Record: Is it Really So Bad? Proceedings of Medical Informatics in Europe, 1994.
[11] Adelhard K, Eckel R, Holzel D, Tretter W. A Prototype of a Computerized Patient Record. Proceedings of Medical Informatics in Europe, 1994.
[12] Herbert I et al. Protocols for Clinical Care. Proceedings of Medical Informatics in Europe, 1994.
[13] Gordon C et al. The DILEMMA Generic Protocol Model. Internal Deliverable of the DILEMMA Project, 1993.
[14] Gordon C. Protocol Task Manager: Functional Requirements. Internal Report for the DILEMMA Project, 1994.

Health Telematics for Clinical Guidelines and Protocols
C. Gordon and J.P. Christensen (Eds.)
IOS Press, 1995

Telematics and Protocols of Care in Critical Care Environments

A J Wilson[a], C L Bowes[b] and J Holland[c]

[a] *IBEES, Lodge Moor Hospital, University of Sheffield, Sheffield S10 4LH UK*
[b] *Kontron Instruments Ltd., Croxley Centre, Blackmoor Lane, Watford WD1 8XQ UK*
[c] *Draeger Medical Electronics, IBC Weg 1, 5680 GA Best, The Netherlands*

Abstract. The paper discusses the potential roles for protocols of care within critical care environments from the perspective of providing real-time support for their application. The discussion is based around a conceptual model of care in critical care environments. This model has been developed in the wider context of developing information technology systems to support clinical care in critical care environments. The conceptual model of care is a three layer model which demonstrates both the hierarchical and temporal aspects of the care delivered to patients. It is proposed that if the value of protocols of care is to be realised in critical care environments then they must be seamlessly integrated into the routine data management associated with the care of patients. In order to demonstrate this and to evaluate the utility of this concept in the clinical environment, the systems from the AIM TANIT (Telematics in Anaesthesia and Intensive Therapy) project have been used as prototype platforms. The application of the concepts developed are described in two critical care environments: the anaesthesia department and the intensive care unit. Problems in using protocols of care in intensive care units suggest that integrating these with a problem solving methodology to create an integrated care plan may be a more appropriate approach to patient management.

1 Background and Introduction

The care delivered to patients in critical care environments is both extensive and complex. Managing the planning and delivery of this care represents a major organisational problem for those working in these environments [1]. One potential way of addressing this problem is to define the care delivered to patients in terms of protocols of care. This paper discusses the possible roles of protocols of care in two contrasting critical care environments and addresses the problems of providing real time information technology support in which protocols of care are seamlessly integrated into the data management requirements for the routine care of patients.

Critical care environments are those wards and specialist units within a hospital where care is delivered to patients who are either critically ill or dependant on artificial organ system support to maintain cardiovascular haemeostasis. Such environments include the general intensive care unit, coronary care unit, post-operative intensive care unit, burns unit, trauma unit and the anaesthesia department. The planning and delivery of care to patients who are critically ill is complex for two reasons: firstly, many different factors need to be taken into account in the clinical decision making process since support for one organ system which is functionally compromised may increase the likelihood of functional insufficiency in another organ system; and secondly, decisions are time critical in that many are made to support a rapidly deteriorating physiological state. Support for the clinical decision making process has already been identified as a key area where support is required in the intensive care unit [2,3].

The use of protocols of care in different critical care environments varies. Of all critical care environments, protocols of care are most widely used in anaesthesia. Protocols currently in use and widely accepted include those for the use of pre-operative X-ray screening, patient monitoring and anaesthetic equipment checks [4]. The composition of many of the protocols is nationally agreed and adherence is driven by the need for quality assurance [5] and medico-legal concerns [6]. It has been suggested that the application of protocols will become more extensive in the future [7]. The use of nationally agreed protocols within other critical care environments is much less common. This is primarily due to differences in the nature of the care delivered, the duration of care and the case-mix of patients treated.

Protocols can exist for all aspects of medical care including admission criteria to the critical care environment, the delivery of care to patients and the use and maintenance of equipment. It is proposed that if protocols are to be of value in the routine care of patients then those associated with the planning and delivery of care must be seamlessly integrated with the data acquisition and recording which is a necessary part of the care of the critically ill patient.

If protocols of care are to become an integral part of the data management supporting the care delivered to critically ill patients, then it necessary to define what "care" is as a precursor to defining the role of protocols within its delivery. This paper proposes a conceptual model of care which describes both the hierarchical and temporal aspects of care in the critical care environment. Based on this conceptual model of care, a role for protocols of care within the overall data management required for patients within the critical care environment is proposed.

The concepts described in this paper have been developed as one component in the wider context of developing information technology systems for critical care environments. In particular, the systems developed within the AIM TANIT (Telematics in Anaesthesia and Intensive Care) project provide platforms for the evaluation of the concepts discussed in the clinical environment.

2 Overview of the TANIT project

The overall aim of the TANIT project is to design, implement and evaluate comprehensive information technology systems in two critical care environments: the anaesthesia department and the general adult intensive care unit. Care of the critically ill requires the collection, storage and retrieval of large amounts of data as an integral part of patient care. The management of this data in a form which easily supports the care of patients is one of the key issues addressed within the TANIT project [8,9]. In addition to the data required for patient care, there is also the data required for the organisational management of the critical care environment. Therefore, the data management requirements for critical care departments can be considered to consist of 2 closely interrelated components:

- A real-time data management component to support the planning and delivery of care to patients.
- A component to support the management of the critical care department including financial management, organisational management and clinical audit

The components of the systems which support the management of patient care are designed to be used primarily in the vicinity of the patient. For the anaesthesia system, this is beside the anaesthetist's work area in the operating room; in the ICU, terminals to the data management system are adjacent to the patient's bed. Both systems have a direct manipulation graphical user interface designed around task analyses of the environments. The systems support the following facilities:

- automatic acquisition of data from patient monitors, ventilators and other bedside therapeutic devices
- entry of manual measurements and observational (qualitative) assessments of patient state
- displays through which patient data can be reviewed
- prescription and delivery of both drug and non-drug treatments
- management of requests for and results from laboratory investigations
- recording of medical and nursing notes

There are two major problems which must be addressed by data management systems aiming to support clinical care in critical care environments [8]: firstly, they must minimise the staff time required to collect and store the data; and secondly, they must present data in a form which optimally supports the clinical decision making process. The approach to the solution of these problems provides the framework for the development of the clinical component of the data management systems. It is into this framework that the support for protocols of care must be seamlessly integrated.

3 Protocols of Care in the Critical Care Environment

As a starting point for considering protocols of care within critical care environments it is necessary to determine what "clinical care" within the environments is. Without some form of principled framework to define this, the role of protocols of care within it are likely to be ill defined. As part of the development work carried out within the TANIT project, a conceptual model of care within critical care environments has been developed. It has been suggested [10] that care can be divided into three hierarchical layers: a "normative" layer, a "strategic" layer and an "operational" layer (figure 1). The topmost layer of the model is the "normative" layer. This layer effectively defines the professional norms which govern the delivery of care. At the very highest level, these are set at governmental level and by the national professional accreditation bodies. These will inform and influence the standards for care delivery set at the level of the local hospital which in turn will inform and influence the standards of care for a particular clinical unit within that hospital. These standards provide, in themselves, protocols of care. As an example of this, minimum standards for patient monitoring are recommended by the American Association of Anaesthetists: this forms a protocol which should be followed in the care of anaesthetised patients. The

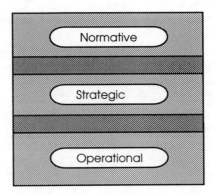

Figure 1: The three layers of the hierarchical conceptual model of care

normative layer is not concerned with tailoring the care to the requirements of an individual patient, but rather with proposing standards of care for the entire patient population.

The middle layer of the hierarchy is the strategic layer. This is the layer in which the care of particular patients is planned. At the topmost level within this layer, are the locally defined standards and guidelines set for the care of patients with a specific clinical problem or combination of clinical problems. At the lowest level within this layer, those involved in the strategic planning of an individual patient's care use the appropriate standards and guidelines to prepare a detailed plan for the care of a particular patient. The process of planning care has two components: the first is assessing the patient's state; and the second is to prepare a detailed plan of care for that patient.

The final layer of the conceptual model of care is the operational layer. In this the strategic plan of care developed in the strategic layer is implemented and carried out. There are several important points to note from the discussion of the conceptual model of care: firstly, although the model is described as three discrete levels it is in practice not made up of discrete layers but is a continuum where the boundaries between the layers are ill defined. Secondly, different players are involved in the decision making process in the different layers of the conceptual model of care. As an example of this: the strategic planning of care in an ICU will be performed by one or more of the senior medical consultants whereas the organising and delivering of that care (the operational layer) will be carried out by the nurses. Finally, the conceptual model of care implies a cross sectional view of care: one in which time is not a factor. This is clearly an inappropriate view since care is dynamic. In practice care involves repeated cycles of clinical decision making (strategic layer) and action (operational layer): the patient state is assessed, a treatment is planned and delivered, the success of that treatment evaluated through observation and measurement of the patient state and the treatment plan modified if necessary (figure 2). The inputs to the assessment of patient state are the normal physiological values, the target values to be achieved with thecurrent treatment regimes (if appropriate) and the current measured values from the patient. The current values from the patient are assessed in the light of the other two sets

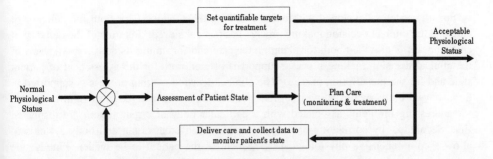

Figure 2: Feedback model of the temporal aspects of care

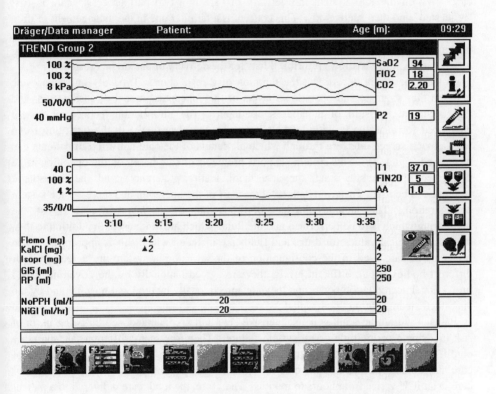

Figure 3: The trend displays and task oriented navigation of the anaesthesia system

of values. If necessary the treatment regime is modified, new treatment targets set and further monitoring of the patient's state continues until the next review of the patient's state occurs. If the current patient state is acceptable, then the cycles of planning and delivering care are concluded. In terms of the conceptual model of care the dynamic aspects of care are represented by repeated crossing of the boundary between the strategic and operational layers. It should be noted that the feedback model for care shown in figure 2 is in itself hierarchical. A single loop of the type shown in figure 2 could be applied to the whole patient. This single loop could then be decomposed into separate loops for each organ and body system for which care is either being administered or potentially required.

For the systems developed within the TANIT project, support for both the delivery of care and the clinical decision making process has been achieved. In terms of the delivery of care, support is provided both for planning the care and for timing its delivery. In terms of the clinical decision making process, support is offered both for the assessment of patient state and for the prescription of care. The clinical decision making process is supported in three ways. Firstly, by providing prioritised data displays in which the most significant data for addressing problems associated with a particular body or organ system are displayed first. Secondly, by correlating data on the state of different organ and body systems to allow a comprehensive physiological assessment of the patient to be made. Finally, the user navigation for the review of patient state is based on body and organ systems. The second part of the support achieved within the TANIT project is support for the timing of care. Within the ICU system the delivery of care is a two part process: care is first "requested" and then "delivered". This concept is a familiar one in the management of drug treatments, but has been extended to cover all care delivered to patients within the ICU. At the time care is requested, target times for its delivery are set. Collating these times for different care requests allows prioritised lists for the delivery of care to be created.

In the anaesthesia department the duration of care is short. Typically only one cycle between the strategic and operational layers of the conceptual model of care occurs: and that occurs at the start of a patient's treatment. The information technology system developed for anaesthesia within TANIT provides the anaesthetist in the operating room with a touch screen interface through which all details of the care delivered to patients can be entered (figure 3). This system supports protocols of care based on the operation to be performed, the patient's state, the anaesthetic team's preferences and the anaesthetic technique to be used. These are entered at the start of the operation and these set the system configuration. This includes the lists of drugs that are displayed in options list, the monitoring which is to be performed and the fluids which are to be used. In addition to this, ranges and typical values for drugs and fluids are included where this is appropriate. The protocols of care used in the configuration of the anaesthesia system are agreed by four different bodies at two different levels: they are agreed nationally by the government and professional accreditation bodes and they are agreed locally by the local hospital and by the anaesthetic teams within that hospital.

Patients within the adult general intensive care unit are characterised by being in, or at risk of, single or multiple organ system failure. Therefore many different, and possibly conflicting guidelines from the normative and strategic layers of the conceptual model of care may be used in planning the care for an individual patient. In addition the duration of care in an ICU varies from hours to months. Therefore, the total care delivered to a patient will involve many cycles of the strategic and operational layers of the conceptual model of care. Within the strategic layer of care, the major tasks which must be performed are the assessment of patient state and the planning and ordering of care. Care in this case includes physiological monitoring, laboratory investigations and treatments. Within the operational layer, the tasks to be performed include validating data from the bedside monitoring, obtaining samples for laboratory investigations, recording the results for laboratory investigations, the administration of treatments and providing general care to the patient. Into this latter category fall such elements of care as turning the patient to prevent bed sores.

It has already been noted that in the anaesthesia department, care occurs over a short period of time and is characterised by a single cycle of planning and delivery. In an intensive care unit, care can occur over a very long period of time and is characterised by repeated cycles of planning and delivery. One other major difference exists between the two environments: in the anaesthesia department, care is planned and delivered by one or a small number of professionals from the same discipline. This contrasts sharply with the intensive care unit where care is planned by many different professionals from (typically) a single discipline, but the total care of the patient is delivered by many professionals from different disciplines. These professionals must co-ordinate their different knowledge and skills to care for patients who are either in or at risk of multiple organ system failure, who have a complex clinical history and whose physiological state is rapidly changing. Within the ICU-Pilot system, it is therefore necessary to seamlessly integrate the support offered for protocols of care with the more general support offered for planning the care of patients (for example a drug prescription screen). It is also necessary to support the working practices of the different professional disciplines who are involved in the care of a single patient. If support for protocols of care is to be accepted as part of the routine working practices of the ICU then a minimum of effort must be required from staff to access and use them. Finally, protocols of care represent measurable standards of care and therefore data should be available to monitor adherence to the protocols as part of clinical audit.   In order to illustrate how protocols of care can be integrated into a real time system for the planning and management of care within an intensive care unit, consider the prototype display shown in figure 4. This screen provides a 'workbench' for the prescription of IPPV. To the left of the panel supporting this are buttons which allow "task oriented" navigation of the system. Above the panel supporting the prescription of IPPV is a panel which normally contains the personal and admission details of the patient. The panel supporting the prescription of IPPV is sub-divided into 5 panes in two columns. The left column of panes contains data entry boxes which allow the prescription information for IPPV to be entered. The majority of ICUs have 'preferred' or 'initial' settings for many of these parameters. These 'preferred' values are site configurable within the system and are displayed when a prescription is first made. Users can edit these values to set the requirements for an individual patient. The values entered are validated against site configurable 'typical' and 'absolute' ranges. If an entered value exceeds the typical range, then a warning message is displayed and the user asked to confirm their entry. If a value outside the absolute range is entered, it is not accepted. These features in themselves, whilst being apparently simple, provide a level of protocol support since they supports local working practices and conventions. The right hand column of panes contain locally configurable lists of measurements and investigations which should be considered when prescribing IPPV.   Those measurements and investigations which are currently being carried out are indicated on the display. The framework behind this method of integrating

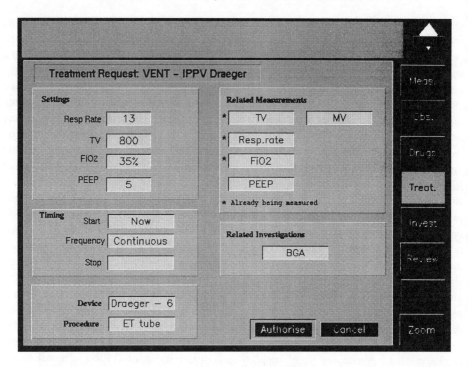

Figure 4: Example screen for prescription of intermittent positive pressure ventilation (IPPV) showing the ventilation parameters. The measurements and investigations displayed should be performed according to the locally defined protocols of care

protocols of care into the overall data management required for the care of patients comes directly from both the conceptual model of care and the case mix of patients treated within an ICU. ICU's essentially provide organ system support for patients in, or at imminent risk of, major organ system failure. Therefore much of the treatment provided in an ICU is centred around supporting failing organ systems. The dynamic element of care within the conceptual model of care is characterised by repeated cycles of assessing the patient's state, prescribing care and delivering care. The patient's state is assessed using clinical observations and the results of measurements and investigations. Therefore, the lists of measurements and investigations provide the monitoring which should be carried out as a result of prescribing IPPV. Such monitoring would normally be specified as part of a protocol of care, therefore the screen shown provides direct support for protocols of care integrated with the overall data collection required for the care of the patient.

Within the anaesthesia department, protocols of care were used to configure the system to the requirements of a particular anaesthetic treatment. A similar use of protocols could be envisaged in the ICU system. Requests for care on admission would be initiated based on the clinical history of the patient and the reasons for admission. This information is normally entered onto the data management system when the patient is admitted to the critical care environment. The complexity of the case-mix necessitates that further work on classifying patients is required for this approach to be widely accepted.

4 Discussion

This paper has proposed a method by which support can be offered through a real time data management system for protocols of care in critical care environments. The need to seamlessly integrate the support for protocols of care into the support for the routine data management required for patient care is discussed. Protocols of care are designed to support the planning and delivery of care to patients. As a starting point for discussing information technology support for protocols of care, a conceptual model of care has been developed which describes both the hierarchical and temporal aspects of patient assessment, care planning and care delivery. Care in critical care environments is characterised by three factors: firstly, it is rapidly changing in response to the changes in the physiological state of the patients; secondly, it is complex in that support for one organ system may well jeopardise the functionality of another; and finally, it is multi-disciplinary. Protocols of care can aid and support the clinical decision making process and can support communication between the different members of a multi-disciplinary team. However the traditional protocols of care, such as those found in anaesthesia, are limited in their application to other critical care environments in that they are essentially rule based definitions addressing only one facet of a multi-faceted problem. One of the driving forces behind the introduction of protocols of care has been as a way of achieving improvements in the quality of care delivered [11], although it is difficult to prove that demonstrable improvements in patient care are a direct result of the introduction of protocols alone [12,13].

The inflexibility in protocols of care is one reason why they have not been widely adopted in critical care environments other than anaesthesia. As an example of this, protocols for ventilation do not consider the age, sex and presence of pre-existing cardiovascular disease [14]. What is perhaps required is a more flexible approach to planning the care of critically ill patients: a framework which supports both the clinical decision making process and the planning and delivery of the resultant care. Such frameworks have been given many names including an "integrated care plan" and a "single patient record". Whatever the name, the most fundamental question is: "what is the functionality and what form should the framework take?" From the discussion within this paper it is clear that it must support the clinical decision making process and it must address the needs of all the different disciplines involved in the care of the patient.

The conceptual model of care described in this paper suggests that an appropriate framework for the integrated care plan would be one based on a problem solving methodology. These are commonplace in other industries and are taught as an essential component of many management courses. Essentially, the patient within the critical care environment has a series of problems or needs which are determined as part of the assessment of the patient's state. These must be addressed and the problem solving methodology provides a logical framework for doing this. A further role of integrated care plans is to address the problem of managing different and sometimes conflicting protocols of care in order to address the problems and needs of the whole patient. This is another aspect of support for the clinical decision making process. Finally, a patient presenting with a complex series of problems and needs will have a long and detailed list of care to be delivered. The delivery of this care requires planning so that it is both optimal in terms of clinical efficacy and causes least distress to the patient. Such support could perhaps be best termed 'prioritising' the care delivered to patients. In critical care environments there is a need to move away from inflexible protocols of care to flexible integrated care plans.

There are few precedents for an integrated care plan, and those which do exist are not appropriate to the critical care environments. Clearly the conceptual model of care and the concepts behind the integration of protocols into the support for routine care of patients are important inputs into the design process for an integrated care plan. Conceptually, the approach of providing support through a problem solving methodology appears an appropriate one, though a great deal of research and prototyping must be carried out before integrated care plans can reach a level of sophistication where they can be evaluated in a clinical environment.

5 Acknowledgements

The work described in this paper is partly funded through the TANIT project (A2036) from the Advanced Informatics in Medicine Programme (AIM) of the Commission for the European Union. The authors gratefully acknowledge the contribution of all members of the TANIT project who have commented on many of the concepts presented in this paper during meetings of the consortium held during the past two years.

6 References

[1]   McNair P, Brender J and Ladefoged S. Impact on resource consumption from application of sequential test strategy. In: Lecture Notes on Medical Informatics: Proceedings of the 9th. Medical Informatics in Europe Conference pp 381-387 Pub: Springer Verlag, Heidelburg ,1990

[2]   Ambroso C, Bowes C, Chambrin M-C, Gilhooly K, Green C, Kari A, Logie R, Marraro G, Mereu M, Rembold P and Reynolds M. INFORM: European survey of computers in intensive care units. Int. J. Clin. Monit. and Comput. Vol 9 pp 53-61 1992.

[3]   Bowes C L, Ambroso C, Carson E R, Chambrin D, Cramp K, Gilhooly K, Groth T, Hunter J R W, Kalli S and Leaning M S. INFORM: Development of information management and decision support systems for high dependancy environments Int. J. Clin. Monit. Comput. Vol 8 pp 295-301 1992

[4]   Taylor D R and Goldhill D R. Standards of Care in Anaesthesia. Butterworth-Heinemann, Oxford 1992.

[5]   Adams A K. Quality Assurance in Anaesthesia. Anaesthesia Vol 30 pp 311-313 1983

[6]   Cohen M M, Wade J, Woodward C. Medical Legal Concerns among Canadian Anaesthetists. Canadian Journal of Anaesthetics Vol 37 pp 102-111 1990

[7]   Baldock C J. Quality assurance, standards and accreditation. Anaesthesia Vol 45 pp 617-618, 1990

[8]   Wilson A J, Molyneux K, Stevens V G, Howes M, Parker-Jones C, Lennard A, Bowes C and Reynolds M. ICU-Pilot: System Design and Preliminary Implementation. Telematics in Anaesthesia And Intensive Care (TANIT -A2036) Deliverable 16, 1993

[9]   Nuijten N and Sclatmann H. Demonstrable Human Computer Interaction Testbed (TANIT - A2036) Deliverable 17, 1993

[10] Friesdorf W. Private comunication. Department of Anaesthesiology, Anaesthesia Technology and Systems Engineering, Steinhoevelstrasse 9, D-7900 Ulm, Germany. 1992

[11] Esichorn J H. Prevention of intra-operative anaesthesia accidents through safety monitoring. Anaesthesiology Vol 70 pp 572-577 1989.

[12] Zeitlin G L. Possible decrease in mortality associated with anaesthesia. A comparison of two time periods in Massachusetts, U.S.A. Anaesthesia Vol 44 pp 432-433 1989

[13] Orkin F K. Practice Standards: the Midas touch or the emperor's new clothes? Anaesthesiology Vol 70 pp 567-571 198

[14] Milic-Emili J. Is weaning an art or a science? Amer. Rev. Respir Dis Vol 134 pp 1107-1108 1986.

Disseminating Quality Care
for Upper Gastrointestinal Cancer

Tim de Dombal and Iain Martin
Clinical Information Science Unit and Academic
Unit of Surgery, The University of Leeds, Leeds, LS2 9JT, England

Abstract. This presentation discusses the problem involved in providing quality care for patients with Upper GI Cancer throughout a healthcare delivery system. It is argued that appropriate telecommunications technology exists for widespread dissemination of "best clinical practice", but that it cannot be used effectively at present because of some limiting factors. These include lack of precisely defined aims concerning use of technology, lack of interactive quality control, and insufficient involvement of end-users. Upper gastrointestinal cancer is selected as a model for discussion - since there is wide discrepancy between outcome of therapy in early and late cases, there is evidence that early diagnosis is possible - and there is substantial evidence that it does not take place widely in practice.

Prospects for the future (with special reference to the 4th Framework) are discussed. It is argued that considerable opportunities exist. Future work should build on existing experience in informatics (eg. the "Telegastro" program) and in clinical practice (e.g. the Leeds "outreach" programmes) for (a) widespread dissemination of effective "best" clinical practice; and (b) continuing medical education.

1 Introduction

Throughout a recent conference at Nijmegen on telematics and oncology in Europe, a major theme emerged; wide agreement (reflected in the pages of this volume) that a principal task in the next five to ten years related to the dissemination of "best clinical practice" - and the need to persuade practising clinicians to follow peer recommended "best practice" guidelines.

This is perhaps the most important challenge of cancer management today - for there is ample evidence nowadays in many clinical areas that the outcome for cancer patients is vastly improved (providing best practice guidelines are followed) - for example in rectal neoplasia where adherence to "best practice" has been shown to influence survival [1]. Unfortunately however there is also evidence that (in many clinical institutions) best practice is not followed. One outstanding example, recently reported from the south east of England, concerns breast cancer [2] where a review of the management of several hundred patients revealed that in over half best practice guidelines had been ignored, and again in over half the patients it was impossible to determine from their case records either the extent or staging of their tumour.

This state of affairs has two undesirable effects. The first is obvious - in terms of less than optimal patient outcome and in terms of less than optimal cost-effectiveness of therapy (for example in breast and rectal lesions). The second is less obvious but no less important to the European Union - for given variety in clinical practices (and patchy, poor, or non-existent data recording), it is clearly impossible to present or evaluate comparisons between centres and institutions on anything other than an empirical basis.

2 Potential Role for Telecommunications

There is a clear potential role for telecommunications in the solution of this pressing dilemma. For if healthcare workers are to follow guidelines, they must first be made aware of them - constantly, on an interactive basis, since it has been shown that the mere dissemination of guidelines does not lead to their being followed. Indeed, there has been much discussion of this prospective role for telecommunications in recent months - not least in the British Medical Journal where the attention of the interested reader is drawn to a leading article entitled "Global Public Health and the Information Superhighway" [3]. These issues are also dealt with in more detail elsewhere in this volume. They will not be repeated here; and are mentioned solely to stress their importance.

3 Telecommunications, Informatics, and Limiting Factors

There are, however, problems.

Given the basic premise that the technology which permits effective communication between different centres now exists, there is need to use it effectively. Unfortunately, this cannot be done at present because of some quite severe limiting factors - and unless these problems are addressed (and overcome) the potentially appropriate technology will not be used to its appropriate potential.

The first of these limiting factors concerns a lack of precisely defined aims. Telecommunications technology works best when it is determined in advance what it is supposed to do - and this is by no means the case at the present time - at least in relation to this particular clinical area. The situation is best epitomised in the remark (quoted by Lee Lusted) [4] by an English Peer of the Realm who when informed one hundred years ago that a land link had been established between England and India and asked to inaugurate it enquired querulously "What shall I say to India?".

Another limiting factor relates to imprecision concerning terminology. If multi-centre studies are to be effective, each centre must use the same terminology and - crucially - each centre must use the same definitions of each term involved. At present, this is clearly not the case - and there is an obvious role for a symbiosis between telecommunications and informatics here, informatics to sort out the imprecision concerning terminology and telecommunications to make the results of these studies widely available. Indeed, the greatest risk of the global superhighway is that the information flowing up and down it will prove to be worthless. This implies the need for a further feature (often conspicuously lacking in multi-centre studies) namely, quality control. This can be achieved using informatics and ideally on an interactive basis, but all too often quality control is ignored - and without quality control over the data, multi-centre studies are open to serious error.

Finally, there is the obvious but often overlooked requirement that the package provided to the end-user should do what the end-user wants it to do! There is clearly insufficient end-user involvement in many current systems; and this, together with the other limiting factors already discussed, has proved a severe handicap to the widespread introduction and effective use of many otherwise admirable telematics and telecommunication systems in clinical medicine. User requirements have been spelt out in detail elsewhere [5]: but two are obviously relevant here. The user must perceive benefit: and systems need to be so co-ordinated that the user does not have to familiarise him/herself twice with two different packages.

4 Why is Upper Gastrointestinal Cancer a Good "Role Model"?

It is the contention of the present authors that upper gastrointestinal cancer forms an excellent model for telematics studies in clinical healthcare. This is so for a number of reasons.

- Upper GI Cancer is a common condition. WHO statistics suggest that up to 15% of cancer deaths world-wide are due to gastric cancer alone.

- Treatment is potentially highly effective. When gastric cancer is detected and treated in its early stages, five year survival rate exceeds 70% in the UK and 90% in Japan [6], [7].

- However, there is strong evidence that this optimal treatment is widely the exception rather than the rule. In many large scale studies five year survival rates have been shown overall to be less than 10%; and the proportion of gastric cancer patients treated at an early stage is similarly low [8], [9].

- Studies from Leeds and elsewhere indicate that the present situation is potentially remediable (at least in part) by the widespread application of good clinical practice. There is a clear link between speed of diagnosis, pathological staging at operation, and subsequent patient outcome. Moreover, studies have shown that it is possible to reduce the "lead time" between presentation and diagnosis (from upwards of 24 weeks to 42 days) by appropriate liaison with primary healthcare [10]. Other more recent studies have shown a concomitant rise in the proportion of patients with early gastric cancer treated over a period of years, this rise coinciding with more aggressive and early use of endoscopy and appropriate surgical therapy.

Studies in Leeds conducted over the past 25 years have shown a rise in Stage 1 gastric cancer from 6% in 1970-74 to over 25% in 1990-94. More than 50% of patients now present with surgically curable disease and the 5 years survival in these patients currently exceeds 60%.

This has been brought about by a 10-fold rise in the number of gastroenterological endoscopies - with consequent earlier diagnosis. Thus both aggressive investigation and treatment can produce nowadays reasonably good results in a disease regarded by many as almost invariably fatal in the West.

- Indeed, one further reason that upper gastrointestinal cancer is a good "role model" is that it could be said that an explanation for the difference in results between Japan and the Western nations has been lack of effective communication - which has not enabled the rapid dissemination of good practice in an East/West direction over the last 20 years.

- Upper gastrointestinal cancer is thus common, it is generally lethal, and there is strong evidence that with the application and dissemination of good clinical practice it need not be so. As such, it is an excellent basis for further study.

TELEGASTRO
Promoting Good Practice via Telematics

*A Suite of Computer Programs Presented by the OMGE
Research Committee and the European Union DG XIII
(Healthcare Education and Telematics)*

OMGE   EC DGXIII

Promoting "Good Clinical Practice"

The Problem

- For the doctor - the clinical medical course is finite, the faculty is finite and the amount to learn has exploded, so it is no longer possible to "know the whole of medicine", even for a single speciality

- For the community - different centres and individuals use different criteria to assess health care, so it is not possible to make valid comparisons or assessments

The Solution

- Secure consensus about "good clinical practice" in specific areas of gastroenterology

- Present compendium of views on "good practice" using TELEGASTRO computer programs

- Distribute widely to young doctors and others

Guiding and Teaching with TELEGASTRO

The Telegastro Suite of Programs

- Cover selected areas of gastroenterology, including acute abdominal pain, inflammatory bowel disease, upper G.I. bleeding, dyspepsia, jaundice, oesophagitis and upper G.I cancer

- Present consensus views on minimum datasets and criteria for diagnosis, extent and severity of disease

- Define terminology used, via a detailed lexicon

- Are flexible and allow the inclusion of local expertise via a 'Local Variants' facility, provide for 'updates', and permit quick scanning and detailed browsing

- Are available in both DOS and Windows formats for wide usage

Figure 1. Main elements of, and rationale for the Telegastro suite of computer programs.

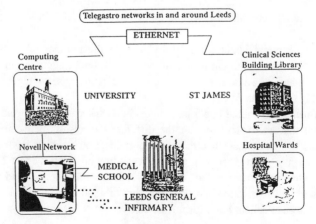

Figure 2. Stylised diagram showing networking arrangements for Telegastro program around Leeds, allowing access by approximately 500 users to date.

5 The Telematics Necessary for Quality Care

In previous paragraphs we have argued that many existing telematics systems have failed because their aims and specification have been imprecisely defined.   We must ourselves now therefore consider the telematics necessary to distribute and promote quality care, (and the feasibility of providing such a telematics system).

In regard to the first consideration, for effective quality care via telematics to be provided clearly a number of conditions need to be fulfilled:-
- There needs to be wide consensus as to what quality care consists of, and how it is to be promoted.
- The terminology surrounding quality care (not least patient entry criteria and end points) need to be widely agreed and clearly defined.
- These considerations need to be embodied into a usable and widely distributable telematics program.
- The program must be capable of embedding in a network, and of use at remote sites by relatively untrained users.
- The program must not merely announce "best clinical practice" but include measures to promote its use at the end-user site.
- Clearly it follows the program must be capable of being networked widely.
- The programs must thus teach and guide as well as inform; and they should contain some kind of interactive quality control over the data entry procedure in participating centres.
- Participating centres must be able to see immediate and tangible benefit if accurate and continued use is to be obtained.

6. Is Such a Telematics System Feasible?

Indeed, it is.   In the last five years, the "Telegastro" system (developed with the support of a grant from DGXIII under the AIM Healthcare Telematics program) has developed just such a telematics product. Wide consultation with clinical colleagues has resulted in consensus of views about "best clinical practice" and this has been converted into a telematics product in three parts:- (a) setting out the clinical consensus of views about best practice, (b) allowing data entry using the above consensus, with interactive quality control, and finally, (c) containing an additional suite of teaching programs to promote interest in the product and interest in best clinical practice (Figure 1).

Additional evaluation has demonstrated the ability of this program to be embedded in local hospital networks and also to be accessed remotely via networks such at Ethernet. Indeed, (Figure 2) the whole of the University of Leeds campus at its varying sites is now capable of accessing this particular program; and there is in principle no difference between an access distance of 2 kilometres and an access distance of 2,000 kilometres.   In theory therefore all the elements to promote "best clinical practice" in upper GI cancer, and (crucially) to impact favourably on patient outcome are in place.

7 Further Studies and Prospects

To sum up, there now exists, in relation to upper gastrointestinal cancer strong evidence that best clinical practice improves the quality of care and patient outcome: together with a proven network for its distribution and for data exchange.   This has authoritative end-user involvement (via the Telegastro project, the World Organisation of Gastroenterology, and National Societies) with virtually every major end-user organisation in Europe.   The program allows precision in data recording (plus on-going quality control) and has many attributes necessary for widespread networking - not least the proven ability of untrained users to put the relevant data on the screen in seconds rather than minutes.   The question arises, what should next be done with this program?

This is perhaps best answered by recalling the needs of oncology in general (defined earlier) - namely (a) precisely defined aims of a network, (b) precision concerning terminology, (c) interactive quality control, and (d) sufficient authoritative end-user involvement.   Proposed studies (possibly within the 4th Framework) thus immediately suggest themselves.

First, there are studies related to the network itself.   There is at present a lack of information concerning "grass roots" use of this type of networked clinical information.   These studies relate both to the technical use of the network itself and to its performance in the hands of well-disposed but relatively untrained (and *very* busy) users.   The Telegastro/upper GI cancer module would seem an obvious potential test-bed for such technical studies (possibly involving the Eurocode network of EORTC).

Secondly, there need to be continuing collaborative studies to define and optimise the definitions of the terminology to be used.   This does not apply particularly to upper gastrointestinal cancer (it is inherent throughout oncology), but the studies are none the less important. Indeed the fact that resulting data are generalisable increases rather than diminishes their value.

Third, the existence of authoritative consensus views and the means to disseminate them clearly offers educational opportunities.   Continuing Medical Education is a major topic at present throughout the whole of medicine.   There seems a golden opportunity offered by the present situation to conduct education studies - possibly using one further section of the Telegastro program (the "GI View" suite of programs provided by the World Organisation of Gastroenterology for this purpose).

Finally, and perhaps most important of all, the answer to the question "What should be done with this network?" should be turned back to the relevant end-users and associated clinicians.   For the bottom line in respect of all of these studies is a simple consideration - the most effective use will be made by end-users who are doing what they want to and using the package and system for purposes which they approve.   There needs to be therefore, strong outreach to the eventual end-users - to find out what exactly they do want and how this package can be made most appropriate to their perceived needs.

References

[1]   McArdle CS and Hole D.   Impact of Variability Among Surgeons on Post-operative Morbidity and Mortality and Ultimate Survival. *BMJ* (1991) 302: 1501-5.

[2]   Chouillet AM *et al.* Management of Breast Cancer in South East England. *BMJ* (1994) 308: 168-71.

[3]   LaPorte RE *et al.*   Global Public Health and the Information Superhighway.   *BMJ* (1994) 308: 1652-
      3.
[4]   Lusted LB.   Introduction to Medical Decision Making.   Springfield Illinois.   C.C.   Thomas.   First
      Edition 1968.
[5]   Zoltie N.   Towards Objective Medical Decisions with the aid of Knowledge Based Systems: Clinicians'
      Requirements.   A Pragmatic Operational Viewpoint.   *Technology and Health Care* 1, (1993) 85-7.
[6]   de Dombal FT *et al.*   The British Society of Gastroenterology Early Gastric Cancer/Dysplasia Survey:
      an Interim Report.   *Gut* (1990) 31: 115-20.
[7]   Maruyama K *et al.*   Progress in Gastric Cancer Surgery in Japan and its Limits of Radicality.   *World J
      Surg* (1987) 11: 418-25.
[8]   Cassell P and Robinson JO.   Cancer of the Stomach: A Review of 854 Patients.   *Br J Surg* (1976) 63:
      603-7.
[9]   Allum WH *et al.*   Gastric Cancer: A 25 Year Review.   *Br J Surg* (1989) 76: 535-40.
[10] Macadam DB.   A Study in General Practice of the Symptoms and Delay Patterns in the Diagnosis of
      Gastrointestinal Cancer.   *J R Coll Gen Pract* (1979) 29; 723-9.

Acknowledgements

The Telegastro program is a telematics product resulting from collaboration between the World Organisation
of Gastroenterology Research Committee Survey Team, national societies and networks, and the AIM
(Healthcare Telematics) programme of DG XIII of the European Union Commission.   This support is
acknowledged with gratitude.

Knowledge Engineering and Methodology

Guideline Based Care: The Challenge for Knowledge Based Decision Support

Pedro Barahona

Universidade Nova de Lisboa and UNINOVA, 2825 Monte da Caparica, Portugal

Abstract. The EPISTOL action was included in the accompanying measures of AIM '91 - '94 as a strategic study, aimed at clarifying the impact in the near future of knowledge based systems and techniques for the health sector, and provide recommendations with respect to the research and development work required within this period. In all the EPISTOL events, namely the Munich and Brussels workshops, the topic of clinical guidelines and protocol and based care raised considerable interest. This paper summarises these discussions, focussing on the KBS support for clinical guidelines.

1 The EPISTOL Action

To aid the planning of future programmes in Health Telematics, in particular the fourth Framework Programme of the Commission of the European Communities and the German MEDWIS Programme, the EPISTOL action was included as a strategic study in the accompanying measures of AIM '91 - '94, based on a contract between the CEC and UNINOVA. The study aimed at clarifying the impact, in the near future, of knowledge based systems and techniques (KBS) for the health sector, and provide recommendations with respect to the research and development work required within this period. The planning of this action encompassed a number of phases and events, briefly described below.

A core group of specialists was appointed which consisted of six invited experts representing research, users, and industry plus the convenor from UNINOVA. Most of the members represented AIM projects or have some other connection with the AIM programme. The main task of this group was the preparation of a Scenario Report with a vision on the future use of knowledge based systems in the healthcare sector, and recommendations about the research and development that needs to be done in this period.

The scenario report was presented at a three days working conference organised in Munich by the MEDIS Institute in 28-30 June 1993. The meeting was attended by the core group, and by over 20 invited experts, representing research, industry, service providers, users, administration and the legal aspect. During the morning sessions of this workshop the convenor presented the Scenario Report and each expert presented a short paper with his/her own vision of the future. In the afternoons, the participants were divided in 4 specialised working groups, each with a specific topic but with multidisciplinary participants. The following topics were discussed: 1) The Role of KBS in Clinical Practice; 2) How Will KBS Techniques Be Incorporated into Commercial Products; 3) Trends in KBS Research that Will Enable Its Use in Routine Applications; and 4) Distributed KBS and Telematics in a Changing Healthcare Environment.

An invitation was widely distributed for participation in an open seminar, held in Brussels in the 19th of November 1993, chaired by the CEC. People expressing interest in participating received the draft scenario document and were requested to submit a short position paper with comments in advance of the seminar. At the seminar the core group presented the revised Scenario Report, the rapporteurs from the working groups of the Munich workshop presented the groups' findings and a member of the core group presented an extract from the 20 plus papers of the same workshop. Following these 8 - 9 speeches a panel with the members of the core group was the centre of a general debate for the rest of the day.

In all the EPISTOL events, namely the Munich and Brussels workshops, the topic of clinical guidelines and protocol and based care raised considerable interest during the events' discussions [1, 2, 3]. This paper summarises these discussions, focussing on the KBS support for clinical guidelines. A more detailed report on the discussions and conclusions of the EPISTOL study can be found in [4], the main deliverable of the study.

This paper is structured as follows. The following section discusses a number of problems that have hampered the dissemination of knowledge based decision support in the health sector, and why supporting the development and maintenance of clinical guidelines is an interesting topic for future KBS research and development. Section 3 discusses a number of issues regarding the modelling and representation of clinical guidelines, and relates them to the modelling and representation of electronic patient records. Section 4 presents a number of challenges for reasoning with these guidelines, and areas where further KBS research and development is required in the near future, and section 5 summarises the main conclusions.

2 Knowledge Based Decision Support and Clinical Guidelines

A main motivation of EPISTOL was the small degree of impact to date in the health sector of knowledge-based decision support, despite the number of useful and proven techniques that KBS research has produced over the years to cope with medical problems. During the various EPISTOL meetings this problem was discussed in great detail.

A great consensus was reached about one main cause of these situation: by and large, there is a lack of integration between medical practice and the knowledge based decision support systems (KBS) that have been developed. This lack of integration can be regarded from several complementary perspectives: the user interface, the communication with other information systems, and the functionality provided.

There is a clear user interface problem with most existing KBS. The interaction with the user is cumbersome and time consuming (e.g. the user has to type in too much data) and this prevents a routine use of KBS. This is possibly one of the strongest reasons why the most widely used KBS to date are in the domain of ECG interpretation. They are hidden inside ECG equipment and require little interaction with the user to produce interpretations of the ECG signals.

Of course, user interfaces have been greatly improved over the last years, and most of the past problems are technically solved or nearly so. Primitive character-based user interfaces have been replaced by much more friendly graphic interfaces based on windows, icons and mouse. Current technology is already enabling the use of multimedia interfaces where these graphic capabilities are extended towards the handling of signals, images and sound, thus removing much of the technical limitations of past user interfaces. Moreover, a number of computers already exist that are able to accept (albeit still in a limited form) handwritten or spoken input, which eases and speeds up dramatically the process of data entry.

Most KBS have been developed in isolation, as standalone systems, which makes their communication with other information systems (and medical equipment) used in the health sector quite problematic, if not impossible. As such, the KBS has no access to the information stored in these systems, and the data required for the KBS, although possibly existing in the information system, has to be re-entered time and again.

Standalone systems have another important and unsatisfactory effect on the user interaction paradigm, as they enforce an "oracle mode" interaction [5]: the user enters the data and the problem to be solved and the KBS provides one or more solutions. Despite all the arguments that KBS may provide explanations to justify the solutions reached, and notwithstanding the importance of these explanations, the fact is that users are distracted from their routine activities into the use a different system, and this is usually not acceptable.

Nevertheless, computers are already in routine use in many health environments, and not only by clinicians. For the moment, their use is mostly aimed at administrative tasks, but some clinical data is already present in these applications. It is thus possibly more acceptable to healthcare professionals to add some decision support functionality into the already existing information systems. These improved systems would thus be regarded by these healthcare professionals as easing their workload (and improving its quality), rather then increasing this load by imposing the use of yet another system.

Of course, the feasibility of this approach is tightly related to the tasks where decision support is provided. Unfortunately, there seems to be a lack of integration between users needs and the functionality most usually provided by medical KBS. Whereas the work in the latter field has been focussing on diagnosis (a highly stimulating research activity), the needs of the users (clinicians and others) are more concerned with global patient care and resource management [6].

In this context, during the EPISTOL activities it became apparent that the focus of KBS research and development should be somehow redirected from simple tasks such as diagnosis into more general planning of patient care, involving not only diagnosis but also treatment, monitoring, etc.

Another problem that has hampered the dissemination of KBS in the health sector is the credibility of the KBS knowledge. Usually, these systems are developed with the aid of an expert in the domain, their competence is usually tested in a significant number of test cases, but their thorough evaluation in clinical trials are seldom performed (usually due to lack of resources). As such, and despite the explanation facilities they provide, the solutions suggested by a KBS are often regarded with a high degree of suspicion by other clinicians.

Given this context, it is easy to see why the topic of guidelines and protocol based care came naturally to the discussion in the EPISTOL events. On the one hand, and despite the fact that there is some ambiguity on what the terms actually mean [7], clinical guidelines and protocols are basically care plans, which largely encompass the whole clinical activity. As such, supporting the development and management of such guidelines is likely to get significant interest from a variety of healthcare professionals, and this interest has already been perceived in some countries (e.g. USA, UK, Holland [1, 2, 8, 9]).

Moreover, they are being strongly supported by a number of important institutions, including health authorities which are seeking ways of containing ever growing healthcare costs, while still maintaining the quality of care. More interestingly, they are being supported by medical societies and other authoritative bodies, which aim to identify sound clinical practice [2, 10]. As such, the above mentioned problem of validating medical knowledge is greatly simplified, when this knowledge is provided by such authoritative bodies, based on a variety of credited sources (experience, literature, clinical trials, etc. [7]).

It would seem that all interested parties should benefit from clinical protocol development and work flow generation from such protocols. The patient can expect to receive a standard of care judged by consensus as being appropriate and to receive that care in a structured and efficient manner. The healthcare professionals should benefit by being able to easily apply the techniques of clinical research to medicine as a whole, and by having access to current "best practice". The healthcare system should benefit by minimising wasteful use or under-use of expensive human and capital resources and thus be able to deliver more care for a given budget.

3 Modelling of Clinical Guidelines

Clearly, the KBS support of guidelines will require the ability to represent their knowledge content. This representation can be regarded at the instance level (i.e. a specific protocol to be applied to a specific patient in a specific environment) or at a more generic level (i.e. a general guideline, and/or a partially instantiated guideline where much of the fine details, such as the exact timings of the actions or a number of alternative treatments are left open). Clearly, the critical issues of sharing and reuse of (medical) knowledge favour the latter approach.

This approach requires of course a structured modelling of the medical concepts involved. This structuring should support the basic concepts of state (e.g. the state of a patient) as well as tasks and actions (e.g. medical acts) and the relationships (causal or other) between actions and state changes. Tasks and actions should be broken down into their components (e.g. simpler tasks) and related to other concepts such as the agents that perform them, the individuals that are subject to them and the objects used to perform them. Moreover, their goals (e.g. measuring a state or changing it) should be explicit, as well as their justification (the knowledge source, including its authoring, and the reasoning that justifies that the goals are indeed achievable).

As care plans, the support of guidelines require that their representation can cope with the timing of the component actions. This representation should therefore include some form of sequential and parallel operators to relate the various actions of a guideline, possibly tagged with some quantitative temporal information (an action should be performed at a specified time interval time after another). Conditional and iterative operators are also necessary to model guidelines with some generality.

The explicit representation of the resources used has an important consequence: the possibility of assessing the resources required by patients following clinical guidelines, and the time when these resources are required. As such, this is an important link between clinicians and other healthcare professionals, since the management of these resources (e.g. the scheduling and optimisation of resources such as hospital beds, drug inventories, etc.) usually involves the latter professionals.

In addition, the explicit representation of the agents of the clinical acts has in turn an important impact on shared care and in the coordination of the care team, and this is of course of paramount importance in a telematics environment. The various agents such as

GPs and specialists, but also nurses and clerical staff can be coordinated by a plan that directly specifies who the various agents are, and when are they required.

This concern with modelling the business structure of healthcare structure is of course already present in many approaches to the architecture of medical records. Indeed, the respective lines of research into generic methods of guideline representation and medical records representation should be somehow concerted, given their complementary nature: a medical record should include care plans (e.g. guidelines applicable to a patient), while a guideline is composed of a number of acts that should eventually be recorded into a patient record. Moreover, the impact of knowledge based decision support in guideline supported care is highly dependent on the availability of electronic medical records. Unless there is a timely access to patient information (for those authorized to inspect them), there is little chance of effective compliance with the care plan specified by some clinical guideline.

In the AIM Programme the need for concertation has been perceived, and informal contact have been maintained between project DILEMMA (dealing with the modelling of generic guidelines) and projects such as GALEN, GEHR and NUCLEUS that deal with the modelling of medical knowledge and more specifically the modelling of medical records.

4 Reasoning with Clinical Guidelines

The previous section discussed a number of topics regarding the representation of guidelines from a knowledge based perspective, and pointed out the similarities with the modelling and representation of patient records, as this might be regarded from a more conventional database perspective. This section focusses on the more specific knowledge based aspects of decision support for the development of clinical guidelines and the management of protocol directed care.

Regarding the management of protocol directed care, and once a protocol has been chosen for a given patient, it might seem that little reasoning is required: all that is needed is to follow the protocol. Nevertheless, there is some reasoning involved. On the one hand, some kind of temporal reasoning is required to identify the starting of actions, and to raise the corresponding alerts and warnings. If protocols are rigid (and some are indeed so, namely some oncology protocols, and some protocols used for controlled clinical trials) this reasoning is relatively simple. There is little or no uncertainty involved, except perhaps on deciding whether a patient should be put on such protocol, or whether should the patient depart from the protocol at some stage.

However, clinical guidelines are usually more flexible (cf. for example [10]), given the uncertainty of medical knowledge and the different health environments where they are to be applied. These more flexible guidelines have to be adapted to specific patients and regional or local health environments, and this adaptation presents some opportunities to knowledge based decision support and points at directions for further research and development.

An important area of research regards the adaptation of a general guideline into a specific patient care protocol. On the one hand, this involves adapting a general guideline into a specific health environment. For example, the exact timing of the different medical acts, such as consultations, may depend on local routines in cases where they are not fully specified in the initial guideline. On the other hand, there are specificities regarding the patient. Some of the treatments included in the guideline may be inappropriate for the patient (e.g. there might be a history of past intolerable side-effects, possibly recorded in the patient record). If the guideline is sufficiently flexible there might be alternative treatments that should be considered (otherwise the patient has possibly to leave the guideline). In any case, and whenever there are many options available, the adaptation of the protocol should aim at optimising some criteria. These criteria include of course patient comfort and other patient related criteria, but also other criteria related to the health environment (e.g. optimisation of the use of resources and overall costs). The assessment of the various options evidently involves reasoning under uncertainty, thus offering potential opportunities for the use of corresponding forms of knowledge based decision support.

All the above adaptations of guidelines will provide opportunities for knowledge based decision support. Since guidelines may be regarded as plan schemes, the Artificial Intelligence work in planning may have much to offer in the required adaptation, namely the work in task management meta-knowledge: the overall organisation of a guideline represents a strategy to accomplish certain goals, and whenever these are made explicit (cf. the previous section), there is an opportunity to guide the decision support process. The work in deep medical knowledge modelling may also be of some assistance, namely to identify implicit interactions between treatments and guide the search for alternatives.

Another KBS research topic quite relevant to guideline support is of course temporal reasoning. This is required in many situations. For example, if the guidelines are flexible enough, the exact timing of the medical acts may be adapted, so that it not only conforms to acceptable clinical constraints but also optimises the use of resources. Also in case of conflicting guidelines, they might be accommodated if the timings of their actions are made "compatible". For example, a certain medication prescribed in one guideline may be postponed until some time after the patient stops an incompatible treatment prescribed in another protocol. Of course, such adaptation is only possible if the goals and rationale of the guidelines and their components are made explicit and a sufficiently deep medical model is made available to the KBS to ground such adaptation.

5 Conclusion

This paper reports on some of the results from the strategic study EPISTOL, regarding the impact in the near future of knowledge based systems and techniques for the health sector. More specifically, the paper discusses the findings related with guideline based care, a topic that raised particular interest during the study.

The paper discusses the reason why the work on supporting clinical guidelines is an interesting topic for medical knowledge based decision support, as it addresses real user needs and poses interesting challenges for knowledge based research and development. Major topics for future research identified in the study, include :-

• Declarative representation of guidelines, where the medical tasks are adequately structured into their composing actions or sub-tasks through appropriate operators (temporal, conditional and iterative), and with an explicit representation of their agents, subjects, objects, goals and justifications.

• Planning and meta-planning research, which is particularly useful whenever the above components are made explicit, and might play an important role in the adaptation of general guidelines into specific patients care plans.

• Temporal reasoning, which regards the sequencing of the medical acts that constitute the guideline, and that might be used, possibly in conjunction with deep medical knowledge, to adapt the guidelines so that they optimise patient comfort, avoid undesired side effects and conflict between concurrent guidelines, as well as optimise the use of resources.

References

[1] A. F. Rickards, D. Pitty and P. Reeves, Knowledge processing and Decision Support in the Health Sector, in [4]: 147-151.

[2] J.-L. Renaud-Salis, Distributed Clinical Management-Information Systems: an Enabling Technology for Future Health Care Programmes, in [4]: 139-146.

[3] E. Coiera (rapporteur), The Role of KBS in Clinical Practice, in [4]: 199-203.

[4] P. Barahona and J. Christensen (eds.), Knowledge and Decision in Health Telematics, IOS Press, 1994.

[5] R.A. Miller and F.E. Mararie Jr, The Demise of the Greek Oracle Model for Medical Diagnostic Systems, Methods of Information in Medicine, 29(1): 1-2, 1990.

[6] J. Wyatt, Routine Use of Medical Knowledge Based Systems, in [4]: 73-79.

[7] D.M. Eddy, Designing a Practice Policy, Standards, Guidelines and Options, Journal of the American Medical Association, 263: 3077-3084, 1990.

[8] J. van der Lei, Computer-based Decision Support: The Unfulfilled Promise, in [4]: 67-72.

[9] A. Farmer, Medical Practice guidelines-lessons from the United States, British Medical Journal, 307: 313-317, 1993.

[10] Guidelines on the Management of Asthma, Thorax, 48 (Supplement): S1-S24, 1993.

A model for the structured description of healthcare activities and related data

A. Rossi Mori, M. De Simone, C. Lalle, F.L. Ricci
Istituto Tecnologie Biomediche, CNR, Viale Marx 15, I-00156 Roma, Italy
Istituto di Studi sulla Ricerca e Documentazione Scientifica, CNR, via C. De Lollis, Roma, Italy

Abstract. Rehabilitation involves long-term, interdisciplinary processes. A model was developed, for the structured description of typical healthcare activities. Telematic services based on this model can support accurate data acquisition and communication among healthcare teams. Presentation of data within their context and according to the specific user's view is envisaged, based on deviations from the typical behaviours. Benefits are also expected in better understanding of the care processes themselves, easier comparison of different approaches, and diffusion of consensus-based knowledge.

1 Introduction

Rehabilitation should be intended as a component of a long-term global intervention — including prevention, appropriate therapeutical actions and social activities — to improve the patient's status, at the maximum level compatible with his/her original impairment [1].

Healthcare provision on individual patients is nowadays shared spatially and temporally among services, which severally contribute to patient-specific integrated programs.

In this context, telematic services should support interaction among healthcare teams, by making available to each team appropriate, timely data and up-to-date medical knowledge, for decisions and actions on individuals, groups, and healthcare services themselves.

The duration of rehabilitation programmes and the number of services typically involved require sophisticated tools to preserve the continuity of the interventions and the proper coordination among independent decision makers.

Here we present a model to describe the set of sub-processes devoted to the global solution of a rehabilitation problem of a patient, based on the formalisation of activities performed by the different actors and the related information requirements, as the way to:

- understand sharing of responsibilities,
- assure coherence of goals among teams, and
- produce a framework for the optimal exchange of information between healthcare

professionals, aimed at patient management and service improvements.

The software applications will use the formalised knowledge and the structured information and data in order to support the professional activity of the healthcare operators.

From protocols to structured care pathways: activities, data, context

Given a medical problem, protocols are ideally the most efficient way to obtain a diagnosis and a therapy based upon locally or more generally reached consensus [2, 3]. Nevertheless, when many actors are involved for a long period on the same patient, it is difficult to formalise all the activities in a very complex protocol, flexible enough to accomodate the features of the available services and the individual variability of the patient's problems and responses. The idea of *"protocol"* (used in biomedical research, multicenter trials, etc.) should evolve into highly flexible and customisable descriptions of the activities performed by a set of healthcare teams. Current protocols will be considered as special cases of the description of an activity, when a short-medium term care scenario is identified; i.e., when a sub-class of patients is defined, with a specific problem and thus with specific care goals.

As a matter of fact, we need a more complex model: flexible, modular, dynamically definable — and re-definable — during its application, able to deal with knowledge, information and data as appropriate during different phases of utilisation [4].

We need also to avoid an overload of detailed descriptions of actions required by each user each user, which are not justified by his/her evolving needs: both the acquisition and the presentation of the "generalised protocol" should be limited at each moment to the minimum necessary for the proper management of the inter-actor communication and to the effective support by computer-based services.

Most detailed data are used for local care provision, and a limited part of this should be carefully selected and made available, when requested, to the other actors. The context in which individual data are acquired and re-used should be formalised and linked to the data themselves, to achieve improved data acquisition acquisition and appropriate use (or re-use).

In part 2 we analyse the rehabilitation environment, in order to work out the requirements for our model of health care activities.

Our solution is presented in part 3; it is based on a modular representation of activities, recursively nested at various levels and with a evolving amount of encapsulated knowledge, information and data. The sub-activities are instantiated, particularised and exploded on request, dynamically supporting the views of the different actors and time windows of different width (a "zooming" effect, ranging from the whole life of a patient to the duration of elementary actions). In part 4 we describe relevant details on the model and its management.

2. Telematic services in shared care: features and requirements

In the rehabilitative field there has, until now, been lacking a global vision of process of the patient, both from a temporal point of view (the sequence of the interventions since pathological event) and from a multidisciplinary point of view (the integration of theraupetic, rehabilitative and social activities performed on the same patient).

In rehabilitative practice the presence of a set of *independent* teams may lead to one of the following situations:

- a sequence of episodic and uncoordinated interventions;
- an improper organisating role of the patient or of his/her family, who tries to coordinate the sub-processes related to the different teams involved;

- a set of well organized interventions over time, due to the leadership of a coordinating team (not pre-organised);
- an integrated programme, based on the reciprocal awareness and pre-organised coordination among the teams.

The optimal situation — the integrated program — is of course very rare: to obtain a really integrated programme, a set of individual plans has to be defined and merged, and applied in a consistent way during care provision.

Telematic services may assist in the preparation, the distribution, the adaptation, the application, and the evaluation of libraries of pre-defined plans, promoting efficacy and satisfaction. Appropriate services may support the proper actualization of a care plan (organisation, monitoring, and synchronisation of activities), improving data collection and exploiting recorded information. In this way they go beyond the mere role of recording information (passive registration of a sequence of Subjective observations, Objective observations, Assessments and Plans).

The impact of these telematic services will vary according to the number of teams that have to be involved on a given pathology and the kind of interaction expected for them.

Therefore it seems appropriate to briefly characterise here some scenarios describing important aspects of healthcare activities.

In table 1 we relate 7 possible organisational approaches of the providers:

1. individual care provider (with loose interactions with other actors);
2. a set of interchangeable care providers in the same organization;
3. a team with various competences and tasks;
4. a set of teams operating "independently";
5. a set of teams allocating tasks between them, in a non pre-defined way;
6. a set of teams operating in cascade;
7. a set of teams operating according to an integrated program.

to a set of 3 descriptive elements:

a. assignment of responsibility;
b. sharing goals and continuity of actions;
c. telematic services.

The 7 organisational approaches of the providers are described here more in detail:

1 - Individual care provider (with loose interactions with other actors)
This scenario deals with an individual healthcare provider carrying out an healthcare related activity on a specific patient. Due to the nature of this activity, there is no a priori need for standardised recording of plans and results. Apart from the minimal legal obligations, the record consists of personal notes.

Table 1. Mapping "main descriptive elements" into "kinds of healthcare provision organisation".
The model of activities in integrated rehabilitation programmes should assist the users in the definition,
management and validation of the common plans, allowing each user to focus on his view being
aware of the context of the others.

main descriptive elements --> *organisational approach of providers*	Assignment of Responsibility	Sharing goals and continuity of actions	Telematic Services
1. individual care provider (with loose interactions)	--	--	--
2. set of interchangeable providers in the same organization	many actors / share among equals	unique goal	*same DB, similar views* updates on patient status / plans
3. team with various competences and tasks	overall leader, chain of sub-responsibles	global goal + subgoals	*same DB, different views* assign - request / report
4. set of teams operating "independently"	many independent actors	autonomous goals	*different systems* isolated messages with synthesis, referral
5. set of teams allocating tasks between them, in a non pre-defined way	coordinating actor, responsible actors and delegated actors	global: unique specific: many	*systematic messaging* referral-request / report
6. set of teams operating in cascade	many actors / similar functions	coherent, evolving	discharge letters, history follow-up plans
7. set of teams operating according to an integrated program	integrated provision, overall "tutor" ?	global: unique specific: many, coherent	common plan as integration of explicit local plans; it relies strongly on telematic services

There are loose and irregular interactions with other providers, that are considered as "services" with very clear interfaces (e.g. general practitioner prescribing drugs or referring to an hospital).

The patient himself ensures continuity of actions among different providers.

E.g.: A patient triggering a specialist visit, or a private dentist treating one of his clients.

2 - Set of interchangeable care providers in the same organization

In this case all the members of the healthcare group carry out in turn the same tasks; obviously, at a higher level, there is a unique responsible for the organization, but each provider is fully responsible during his time-slice. The record should support the continuity of action, even if an additional (oral) update often completes the transferring of responsibility.

E.g.: In a hospital, in order to guarantee the necessary continuity of the assistance of a patient after surgery, monitoring is carried out by the nurse on duty.

3 - Team with various competences and tasks

This involves a healthcare team operating in a given organization according to a chain of responsibilities (e.g.: the physician-nurse relationship). A team member may assign a sub-task to the appropriate team member and receives a report. Every task should be viewed as a step towards reaching a unique goal.

Some of the team members may be separately responsible for a sub-set of activities to achieve a sub-goal (e.g. surgeon vs anaesthetist). The assignments is made systematically or on a case by case basis.

4 - Set of teams operating "independently"

In actual situations, a patient may independently involve different teams (in different moments, without pre-defined agreements among them), each one carrying out a given activity. Some interactions between teams may occur, often accomplished by the patient himself.

Examples of this situation can be found in the life of many patients who need two or more different interventions, not necessarily co-ordinated except through the patient's personal agency.

5 - Set of teams allocating tasks between them, in a non pre-defined way

We may consider a scenario where different teams, perhaps from different organisations, are interacting in a non pre-defined way about the same patient, on the basis of their respective expertise, to achieve a unique general goal. A meta-responsible holds the global responsibility and assigns to a team its tasks and should receive a report.

E.g.: A general practitioner may require for a given patient a specialist's visit or a specific test: the results are reported to him so as to ensure continuity of care.

6 - Set of teams operating in cascade

This scenario deals with a group of teams operating sequentially on a time slot basis; each group must achieve a certain goal that can vary with the time, making necessary the intervention of a different team. Interaction between teams is discrete, occurring probably only when the responsibility is passed.

E.g.: A patient suffering from an evolving pathology may be taken in charge by different teams in sequence.

7 - Set of teams operating according to an Integrated Program

The teams operate according to a pre-defined integrated program: the interventions may fully or partially overlap and the *interaction is continuous* and controlled on a more programmed basis.

Explicit plans of the activities of each team will contribute to the shaping of a common plan.

It is important to stress that, in real situations:
- the scenarios described are not exclusive;
- each interaction between individuals or teams implies information flows;
- the coexistence of different individuals in a team - and of different teams - implies assignment, sharing or transfer of responsibility (both from an healthcare and a legal point of view).

To support telematic services within an integrated program, the description of activities should be re-usable, parsimonious, flexible in time, and customisable according to resources and patients.

Moreover, the description should support the following features:
- it cannot impose a behaviour on a team, unless spontaneously accepted;

• in principle, it should provide an escape mechanism (with possibility of storing the motivation of the deviation for subsequent analysis), for permanent adaptation to the local situation (resources, habits, policy, school), or for case-based exceptions;

• it needs to be pragmatically adaptable to evolving real situations (with the management of expected or unexpected events that influence the process, during execution of a plan, such as patient co-morbidity, unavailability of devices, etc), even if out of the control of healthcare operators;

• it needs to support the co-presence of many processes that are simultaneously "open" on the patient, even if they don't operate at the same moment on the patient (e.g., sets of sessions, sequences of follow-up visits, drug therapies), and of activities whose order is not predefinable (e.g., a set of assessments by different specialists, that are scheduled according to their availability).

If a set of pre-defined care plans is prepared by authoritative bodies, suitable for a class of situations (classes of patients, pathologies, problems), a set of questions will arise:

• where and when is a specific care plan exactly applicable ?
• in which context ?
• who is responsible for what ?
• how and when will the care plan be used ?
• what data are tipically available or produced in a given situation ?
• what kind of interactions with other professionals are expected ?
• are two situations similar?
• are potential solutions similar? (organisation, resources, actors)
• how to select appropriate cases for design/evaluation?

A proper structured description of the care plan — according to a precise model — will facilitate the answering of these questions.

3. Dynamic encapsulation of knowledge, information and data

Our model is based on a modular representation of processes. Each module is recursively nested in a more general module, that also represents the context for its proper use: we may think about each step as a layer providing the *context* for the lower layer.

Organisation of a care plan in a "Context Tree"

Activities and their recursively nested sub-activities are thus organised in a tree, which we call a "context tree" [5]. A library of generic modules — a knowledge base with formalised knowledge describing the typical activities at the different levels of complexity — should be produced and made available. The users will select from the library the relevant modules, compatible with specific services and patient classes.

Given a specific patient, the appropriate modules are gradually selected, instantiated and exploded to dynamically create a patient-specific context tree. Actual patient data enables the modules on the description down to the most elementary activities to be instantiated and exploded, to assist actual care provision (see table 2).

The most general module of a pathology protocol is named the "Life Long Program" (LLP); a generic lower-level module may be re-used in different positions of an LLP and in different LLPs.

Table 2. Influence of constraints on the particularisation of parameters in a description.

constraints --> effect on:	none (as in the library)	on service	on patient problem (protocol)	on planned provision (agenda)	after provision (history)
patient	theoretical	theoretical	theoretical / class	real	real
actors, methods, devices	class	specific class, list of individuals	specific class, list of individuals	identification of the individual	identification of the individual
choices	open	partially defined	defined/some excluded	defined/partially decided	decided
time	generic as arrangement and possible range	generic as arrangement and possible range	constrained by synchronisation among defined activities	scheduled: appointments and agenda	performed: time of actual provision
clinical and organisational data	field name + admissible values	field name + compatible values	field name + compatible values	field name + expected values	field name + actual values

The Life Long Program may be defined as: "the evolving model to express a structured set of activities planned or performed on a specific client, from the awareness of a problem to a complete remission of the consequent handicap or to an appropriate follow-up".

Given a patient in a service, an instance of the related LLP module is activated. At the beginning, when the LLP is copied from a library, it contains mainly knowledge and its sub-activities are not yet instantiated or exploded. The knowledge encapsulated in an LLP is not static, but evolves during time according to the evolution of the status of the client, resulting from the interaction of two processes: the pathophysiological process producing the impairment, and the care process attenuating it.

The LLP module specifies which sub-activities are typically involved, which are the typical actors, devices, etc.: by selecting the appropriate modules which describe specifically constrained sub-activities, or by the specialisation of parameters in the descriptions, the care plan is gradually adapted to the service and the patient class.

By exploding in turn the sub-activities, according to the running constraints of the status of the patient and the availability of resources, the individual care plan becomes more and more specific. The same structure can encapsulate the actual information of the agenda, and can act as the context for the data that are acquired in consequence of the care provision.

During an individual health care process, each instance (and the modules nested inside it) follows its own life cycle [3]; the transition features and the compatibility of six statuses in activities and sub-activities were studied: **performed, operative, scheduled** and **planned**, together with **cancelled** and **suspended**.

On the basis of the above structure, we may obtain the representation of the past, the present and the future of a given patient's LLP at a specific moment (see fig.1), respectively as:

• patient history (the past), i.e. a view organised according to performed activity modules;

• agenda (the present), i.e. the activity modules scheduled in a given moment;

• plan (the future), i.e. the activity modules to be performed and compatible with the context, at different level of detail (and different scope in time).

While the cumulated patient history and agenda are incrementally well defined, the plan is a dynamic programme, adequately and timely specified, never a rigid and complete plan.

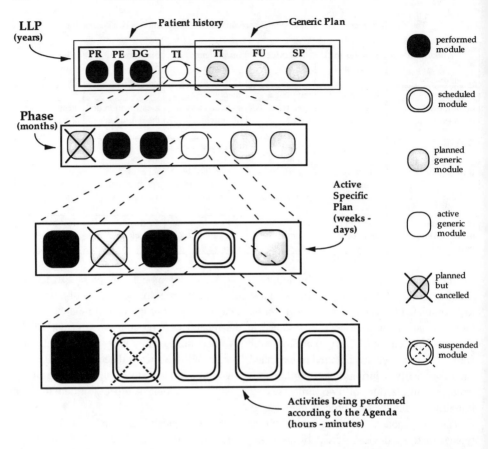

Fig.1 - Modular representation of processes according to the model of activities in Context Trees (typical width of the temporal windows for the activities at each specification level are specified)

The plan is a programme built up step-wise from modules, having an active Life Long Programme as framework and extending down to the actual provision of care by organizing the sequence of phases according to patient evolution, then defining specific care plans, down to the elementary actions.

At a given moment, the construction of a plan covers the scope of the foreseeable future, i.e., until the next major decision or expected event. Moving away from the present, the plan turns to be relatively vague, in time and in potential actions to be performed.

The zooming effect due to the tree organisation may be exploited to browse the knowledge in a generic LLP not yet instantiated, to customise an LLP to a service or a subclass of patients, to guide the consultation of the agenda and of the future plan on a specific patient, or to select and organise historical data about a set of clinical cases.

4. Synergic and semi-structured representation of activities

An activity, according to our model, is described by the following kinds of knowledge:
- frame-based description, exploiting terminological ("kind-of") hierarchies;

- nested scripts on sub-activities and interrupt-based synchronisation with other activities;
  - forms for data I/O, including process variables (execution status);
  - maintenance (author, version, references, validation status, etc).
In the following of this paragraph we discuss in detail the previous items.
Frame - based description
The basic structure of an activity is shown in table 3 according to a frame-like schema. Slots can be multiple and with sub-slots.

The domain of potential values for each slot is organised into a kind-of hierarchy, from the terminological point of view. For example, a possible list for "Actor" may be:

```
Actor
    healthcare provider
        clinician
        nurse
        ...
    client
    family
    relatives and friends
    skilled volunteers
        ...
```

This allows to cluster the descriptions into "families" of similar activities, and their step-wise specialisation.

All the entries express the appropriate (default) values for the specific activity, and can be replaced by more specific ones or unique identifiers at the different steps of instantiation. For example, the value "orthopedist" can be refined stepwise to:

- "pediatric orthopedist", when the age of the patient is known,
- the list of the pediatric orthopedists working in a given service, when the unit is known, and
- the name of the actual physician, when the appointment is given.

Table 3. Frame - based description of an Activity

- is carried out by	Actor			
		which	belongs to	Team
			works in	WorkingPlace
			has additional role	{responsible, contact, tutor}
			uses	Device
			refers to	Community
			has visibility	{yes, no}
- is carried out in	Location			
- is carried out according to	Method			
- is carried out on	Target			
		which	presents Problem	
- aims at	Goal			
- has total duration	<duration value>			
- is made of	sessions			
whose frequency is	<frequency value>			
each is active during	<duration value>			

One or more actors, *visible* or not by other activities, contribute to the activity. An actor may have different additional roles: the responsible within the team, the contact towards external activities, the contact towards the patient (tutor). The actor may have preferences about how to fill out the detail of the sub-activities under his/her responsibility, deriving from his/her membership of a specific cultural, professional or linguistic community.

The *target* can be typically the patient or the family.

An activity is "active" for a specified contiguous interval of time, during which different sessions can be performed.

Nested scripts on sub-activities

An activity is divided, recursively, in typical sub-activities. The typical link among the subactivities is normally homogeneous within an activity, and we have experienced the following kinds of links:

- the sub-activities should be activated in the exact temporal sequence as listed;
- the order is decided during provision (event-driven or user-defined), by simple, specified conditions
- the order is irrelevant;
- the sub-activities are activated together (co - scheduled);
- the order depends on variables which appear in a simple flow - chart;
- the decision is very complex:
- completely managed by the user;
- suitable for a decision support system.

The most frequent case is that all sub-activities should be performed; sometimes there is a selection, and it is relevant to formalise the appropriate run-time constraints: on total duration; on total number of similar sub-activities (e.g., exercises); on total costs, etc.

The typical phases that we have encountered may be organised according to the following classes; the assessment may involve a specific activity, or it is performed implicitly in most cases:

- [self trigger]
- [confirm triggering, from available data]
- avoid start (counter indications / prerequisites)
- assess_before
- [confirm plan]
- perform + assess_during
    prepare
    do
    close
- assess_after
- follow up

The "assess_during" sub-activity is a continuous evaluation of pre-defined parameters, which may generate an internal interrupt. An interrupt may also arise from pre-defined external events, that are known to interact with the activity. The interrupts should be managed according to specific scripts, which involve the following typical actions:

- continue (ignore)
- pause
- resume
- close gracefully
- exit immediately
- stop this activity and activate another activity instead
- continue and activate another activity in parallel
- pause this activity ; activate another activity, and at its completion resume this one
- merge with another activity, yielding a new one

Some scripts require the formalisation of specific modules, describing the activities to be performed when a set of conditions are satisfied (for example replacing two independent activities by a combined description of their interaction). Note that also the "ignore" value is relevant, to process correctly the expected influence of a given interrupt on a specific activity.

Data generation and use

An activity can generate, use, or modify data. Data may be "visible" by other activities (influencing decisions in a following moment) or only "internal" (used during provision for the management of the activity, perhaps recorded for legal purposes only).

Data belong to a structured collection (e.g., database record, message, screen form) and may be split dynamically into field + value, according to the specific implementation of the collection:
   - "fields" are described by the model / structure of the collection;
   - "values" are the actual content of the collection.

The process variables produce intrinsic data, defined for every activity:
- execution status of the activity (planned, suspended, performed, ...)
- instantiation status of slots; for each slot:
   - the value is still as generic as in library;
   - the value is more specific than in library (but not uniquely identified);
   - the value is uniquely identified;
also with reference to calendar time, patient file, other activities.

Maintenance (author, version, references, etc)

This kind of knowledge is not only for documentation purposes, but also to ensure awareness of the source of the encapsulated knowledge, and the reliability of that knowledge (validation, consensus, etc.).

At the moment of explosion of subactivities, more than one alternative description may be compatible with the protocol, and therefore, taking account of the cultural distance between the author and the user, it should be possible for the user to select the most appropriate description given the user's preferences and cultural communities.

5. Discussion

The model we presented above provides different layers of application.
The first layer is about cooperative formalisation and diffusion of validated *knowledge*: the model provides a basis for a methodology and related telematic tools for initiatives in:
- design of care plans
- validation of care plans
- agreement and consensus on a care plan
- training and diffusion of updated and authoritative care plans

In our experiments, the formalisation made it possible to discover analytically:
- the weak points in a plan,
- the disagreements and the points of view in similar plans by different authors.

In the *information* layer, the detailed awareness of information needs of the other actors allows a better (computer-assisted) acquisition, aimed at re-use of data in different explicit contexts; two initiatives are needed here:
1. clarify the human-to-human interaction, in order to get the relevant information and appropriate details, together with their context, suitable for the proper support of the actions of various actors;
2. enhance the human-computer interaction; not so that the computer will provide to the physician rigid advice on what to do, but so that it can act as an intelligent support for professional activities: let the computer "understand" what the physician is (normally) doing, in order to predict his care process and provide more friendly and active interfaces.

In the *data* layer, the approach aims at a reduction in the cost of cooperation. The usual proceess of building the conventional patient history — a serial process with frequent reconstruction of past data — has to be transformed into a parallel process in shared care.
The healthcare professionals are forced to share their data with the other teams that cooperate on the same patients, to make common action possible, and to share responsibilities.
The model offers the possibility to select and aggregate the relevant data, to facilitate the production of notes that are usable for others, not only for the author.

Typical behaviours and actual care provision: checking for deviations

The recursive explosion of subactivities allows formalisation of the default typical sub-activities in the libraries, but also to instantiate at the appropriate moment the description of the sub-activities really used in the care provision. This approach will "transform" a deviation into the timely replacement of a specific module, so that the new module will continue with the correct description. This mechanism allows to monitor carefully the exact points of deviations, for audit or self assessment.
The deviation-based approach allows the amount of information appropriate in context to be delivered; thus the enhanced interface will highlight abnormal or unexpected events data values, contrasting these with typical expected results.

Terminological coherence: the GALEN added value

The present model of activities allows terminological hierarchies relating to actors, devices, problems, etc to be identified and exploited; the management of such hierarchies is a task for the terminological services provided by GALEN (Generalised Architecture for Languages, Nomenclatures and Encyclopaedias) — a project in the EC-AIM Programme.

With the assistance of the GALEN services, it is also possible to:
- create and browse large multiple hierarchies of concepts;
- assure standardisation (for transferability of models and faithfulness of messages);
- manage predefined medically sensible concepts.

The utilisation of the GALEN methodological and application achievements will improve the "terminological" transferability of the formalised modules.

6. Conclusion

The approach here presented puts rehabilitation in a global healthcare perspective. The impact of telematic services on healthcare problems depends on various parameters:
- the perceived need of telecommunication facilities;
- the degree of interaction among actors;
- the usefulness of telematics to improve data collection, storage, retrieval, communication, summarisation;
- the present and possible level of organisation of activities inside a service and among services.

According to our analysis, in the rehabilitation field a complex model of activities is needed, and the impact of this model may dramatically improve the organisation of care.

Our model was at first developed in the IREP Project (Integrated Rehabilitation Programmes), to describe the information and communication needs related to rehabilitation problems (by speciality, by disease, by service, by area, ...) according to the LLP.

It provides an environment for protocols, procedures, care plans, considering them in a continuum:
- from global healthcare goal and context;
- to the implementation of a protocol;
- to the performance of a specific elementary action.

Our work is evolutionary and may undergo extensions every time new disciplines/pathologies are included within the scope of planning, so as to build really "integrated" rehabilitation programmes.

The formalisation is directly exploitable by computer to assist care provision; after customisation, the end-user who is planning or performing an activity will select the proper sub-activities and then will enter or consult data according to the related customised screen; the network will allow relevant data to be made available in a timely manner by and to the other teams.

This model was driven by the needs of the healthcare providers; the final model of the activities, implemented in the future commercial products, should be negotiated — by an iterative process of specification, implementation and evaluation — in order to reach a compromise among:

- the flexibility and the richness of the representation required by care providers,
- the precision and the formal properties needed by software engineers,
- the resources available for future development and implementation cycles, to reach the appropriate level of complexity and usefulness for the end-user.

Acknowledgement

IREP (Integrated Rehabilitation Programs) was a 2 years Project (1992-93) of the AIM Programme (Advanced Informatics in Medicine), partially funded by the European Union (project A2018).

References

[1]   IREP Consortium (avalable from the Main Contractor, TSD Datamont, via Taramelli 26, Milano)
       - Deliverable 1: Overview of Existing Rehabilitation Processes in Europe, 1992
       - Deliverable 2: IREP Process Model - First Version, 1992
       - Deliverable 5: DKB Data Model Specification, 1992
       - Deliverable 9: Global Architecture and Design Guidelines, 1992
       - Deliverable 8: Multidisciplinary Rehabilitation Protocols, 1993
[2]   Gordon C., Herbert S.I., Jackson-Smale A., Renaud-Salis J-L: "Care Protocols and Healthcare informatics" in "Artificial Intelligence in Medicine" Proceedings of the fourth Conference on Artificial Intelligence in Medicine Europe, Editors: Andreassen S. Engelbrecht R. and Wyatt J., Eds. IOS Press, 1993, pp 289-307.
[3]   A.M.Florit, M.De Simone, A.Rossi Mori, A.Patacconi, M.Galanti "The AIM-IREP project on integrated rehabilitation programmes: the IREP vision" in "Proceedings of MIE 93", Eleventh International Congress of the European Federation for Medical Informatics, Jerusalem, Israel - April 18-22, 1993 - Editors: A.Reichert, B.A.Sadan, S.Bengtsson, J.Bryant and U.Piccolo, Freund Publishing House, Ltd., 1993, pp.74-78
[4]   Visser M.C., Hasman A., Van der Linden C.J.: "Protocol processing system (ProtoVIEW) to support residents at the emergency ward" in "Proceedings of MIE '94", Twelfth International Congress of the European Federation for Medical Informatics, Lisbon, Portugal - May 22-26, 1994 - Editors: Barahona P., Veloso M. and Bryant J., 1994, pp. 138-143.
[5]   Florit A.M., Rossi Mori A., De Simone, D'Annunzio V., Ricci F.L., Lalle C..: "Context trees: acquiring knowledge on co-operative healthcare activities in IREP" in "Proceedings of MIE '94", Twelfth International Congress of the European Federation for Medical Informatics, Lisbon, Portugal - May 22-26, 1994 - Editors: Barahona P., Veloso M. and Bryant J., 1994, pp. 618-623.

Health Telematics for Clinical Guidelines and Protocols
C. Gordon and J.P. Christensen (Eds.)
IOS Press, 1995

Prescription Guidelines in OPADE: what are they, how are they used ?

Isabelle de Zegher[a], Claudine Milstein[b], Bertrand Séné[b] and Alain Venot[b]

[a]*BIM, Belgium*

[b]*Eclimed, Paris V University, Cochin Hospital, France*

Abstract. Many computerised drug prescription systems have been developed, but they are rarely used in clinical practice; among the reasons are their lack of integration with the functioning of medical institutions and the lack of consideration of general and local clinical practice rules. We present in this paper how OPADE, a computerised drug prescription system does answer this shortcoming by introducing prescription guidelines called Prescribing Principles. We argue that introduction of these Prescribing Principles will not only allow for integration of the computer in medical practice but will also introduce a positive feed back loop in the prescribing process.

1. Introduction

Computer-aided therapy management has been developed with more or less success for many years. Among the 37 computerised drug prescription systems (CDPS) we evaluated early 1992 [1], one of the shortcomings which appeared repeatedly was the lack of integration and customisation with local medical practice related to prescribing. A direct consequence of this is the limited use of CDPSs by practitioners and their minimal impact on clinical practice.

The aim of the OPADE CDPS is to provide to the prescriber critiques and suggestions allowing him to optimise his/her prescriptions in terms of efficacy, safety and cost. These critiques and suggestions are essentially derived from the evaluation of a patient prescription with three sources of knowledge:

- knowledge relating to a manufactured drug, its composition, administration and regimen, to a pharmacological class or to a pharmacological form; examples are contra-indications, maximum admissible dose, incompatibility in perfusion etc.
- knowledge permitting to infer physiological and pathological states of the patient, which are relevant in the drug prescription context; examples are total body area, renal insufficiency etc.
- knowledge of how to compute prescription costs and reimbursements to the patient.

All three sources of knowledge are essentially in the form of atomic facts and do not provide for linkage betwen the different sources, or for common sense knowledge or rules of clinical practice used within the prescription process. These latter types of knowledge are called in OPADE 'Prescribing Principles' (PP); they convey knowledge from various sources and cannot be attached to the three categories presented before.

In the following, we describe in more details the needs, structure and use of these PPs within a computerised drug prescription system such as OPADE.

The paper is structured as follows. Section 2 provides a description of the rationale for introducing Prescription Principles within the OPADE system. In Section 3 we provide a more complete definition and classification of these Principles; Section 4 contains a detailed description of their internal representation and discusses compatibility with the Arden syntax. In Section 5 we study how these Prescribing Principles can actually ease integration of a computerised drug prescription system in medical practice and we discuss how they could positively influence prescribing behaviour.

2 Rationale for Prescribing Principles

2.1 Description of OPADE

OPADE aims at developing and evaluating an intelligent, multilingual CDPS adapted to different European countries; the system will allow for drug prescribing at the patient bedside in hospitals, or during consultations by general practitioners. An important differentiating factor between OPADE and other CDPSs is that it intends to provide support to the prescriber not only on the medical level but also on the economic and patient compliance aspects.

OPADE is being implemented using a client/server model in which we distinguish three main blocks.

1. The Prescribing Client is composed by the Prescription Kernel and the User Interface; it is the core of the system which manages interaction with the user and evaluates the patient prescription based on the information it requests from the servers.
2. The Data Base (DB) Server handles retrieval and storage of patient and user data needed by OPADE.
3. The Knowledge Base (KB) Server has four components:
   - the Drug KB contains all information on drugs modeled in four levels: active components, generic, manufactured preparation and presentation;
   - the Cost Model KB contains knowledge dealing with computation of cost and reimbursement, validated in different European countries;
   - the State Model contains knowledge used to derive information such as patho-physiological states from a patient's raw data;
   - the Prescribing Principles contain knowledge dealing with prescribing practice rules to be applied within a clinical site.

2.2 The Need for Prescribing Principles

The requirement to introduce the concept of 'Prescribing Principles' within OPADE is illustrated by the following examples, where the system is expected to react with a warning:

1. the physician prescribes tablets for a patient with vomiting, or suppositories in a patient with diarrhea;
2. the patient has to take more than five drugs simultaneously (the same day);
3. the prescribed times of drug intake are not adapted for a night worker;
4. the intra muscular route is chosen for a patient already taking anticoagulants;
5. two drugs containing anti inflammatory substances are prescribed simultaneously to the same patient;

6. in a patient with severe hypertension, the local therapeutic committee advises prescribing a-blocker X and diuretic Y.

The corresponding rules or Prescription Principles needed to identify these potentially 'erroneous' prescription are as follows:

1. Avoid tablets in patients with vomiting or suppositories in patient with diarrhoa;
2. Avoid prescribing more than five drugs for one patient;
3. Avoid prescribing day intake in patients sleeping during the day;
4. Avoid selecting the intra-muscular route in patients with anticoagulants;
5. Avoid prescribing two drugs containing anti inflammatory substances in any patient;
6. Suggest beta-blocker X and diuretic Y in patients with severe hypertension.

Principles 1 and 4 could be contained in the drug knowledge base, in the description of tablets, suppositories and intra-muscular route. For instance, the object tablet could contain the attribute contra-indication with the value 'contra-indicated in vomiting patients', though this is rarely done as such because it involves pure common sense knowledge. The other principles (2, 3, 5,6) cannot be easily included in the drug knowledge base because these are based on various sources of knowledge and involve several medications.

3. Definition and Classification of Prescribing Principles

The considerations of the preceding section demonstrate the need for the introduction in the OPADE Knowledge Base Server of a linkage component conveying knowledge which is not only linked to the drug aspects or patient state or costs calculations, but to all three of them.
From a practical point of view, it is not always clear how to make the distinction between information that should be expressed within Prescribing Principles (PP) or information that should be inserted within one of the other knowledge base components. To make this distinction, we take as criteria that *a PP is an element of knowledge which either links several existing knowledge sources, or is based on knowledge derived from the other knowledge sources*. This definition should be further validated in the light of work currently being undertaken done around protocols and guidelines.

Linking or abstracting various sources of knowledge may happen in several ways and it seems important to clarify this linking mechanism through a classification of the PPs. Within OPADE, we distinguish four categories: logical, rules of thumb, legal and policy constraints.

1. The logical principles have a rational explanation. An example is 'avoid prescribing daily intakes of drug in night workers', or the prescription of drugs and tests for the treatment follow up.
2. The rules of thumb are empirical and consequently cannot be formally validated; they are aimed at modifying prescriber behaviour. An example is 'avoid prescribing more than five different drugs simultaneously'. It seems to be good practice but the number of five is arbitrary and cannot be justified by a logical process, and sometimes five drugs are necessary.

3. Legal rules describe the legal aspects of a prescription such as the type of prescriber allowed to prescribe a given drug or pharmacological class to a certain class of patient, or specification of the format required for the prescription of a drug or a pharmacological class.

4. Rules resulting from policy constraints are principally aimed to decrease wasteful prescriptions and excessive drug consumption which is present in some European countries. An example is "Avoid prescribing some anti-acneic drugs for cutaneous photodamage in women". Other policy constraints can be defined by local therapeutic committees to enforce uniform drug therapy management within the institution. This is the case of Example 6 provided above.

Each type of principle may be the result of an international, national or only institutional consensus. Provision may even be made to allow an individual to enter his/her own PP.

The classification provided above corresponds to the needs identified within the OPADE system; further extension and validation of this classification is needed.

4. Representation of Prescribing Principles

Prescribing principles have four main components:
1. a *patient state value* describing the patho-physiological state of a patient;
2. a *prescriber feature* describing any relevant legal feature of a prescriber;
3. a *prescription feature* which is a synthetic, abstract expression derived from the prescription of one or more drugs; it is built from 5 parts :-
   - a *prescription element* describes one precise element of the prescription; they are qualitative prescription elements such as the name of the manufactured preparation, or pharmaco-therapeutic class, the galenic form, the prescription unit, etc.; there are also quantitative prescription elements such as the number of manufactured preparation or the quantity of prescription unit;
   - a *prescription view* adds temporal conditions on the prescription element; there are three prescription views: whole treatment, per day and per intake;
   - a *optional conditional criterion*, allows additional conditions to be expressed on the evaluation of the prescription element; conditional criteria are themselves composed of a prescription element, an arithmetic or logical expression and a prescription element value;
   - an *arithmetic or logical expression;*
   - a *prescription element value* which is attached to the prescription element.

   The possible combinations of these 5 parts is large but not all of them are meaningful and some could even lead to inconsistent requests; the allowed combinations have been precisely defined with the Prescribing Principle component of the OPADE KB.
4. an *action* which may be either a warning ('avoid') or a suggestion.

These various components, together with additional maintenance information have been structured according to an object-oriented model.

To illustrate the representation described above, we show here how the three first examples as well as the last one of Section 2 can be represented. Another example involving conditional expression ('no more than 2 drugs in drop form can be taken at the same intake time') is also provided.

Component	Example1	Example2	Example3	Example6	Example4
Patient Feature	diarrhoea	any	night worker	severe hypertension	any
PrescriberFeature	any	any	any	any	any
PrescriptionElt	galenic form	number of manuf prep	moment of intake	manufactured preparations	number of manuf prep
PrescriptionView	whole treatment	per day	whole treatment	whole treatment	per intake
CondElt	(-)	(-)	(-)	pharmacotherpautic class = beta bloquant; pharmacotherpautic class = diuretic	prescription unit = drop
ArithLogExpr	=	>	=	=	>
PrescEltValue	tablets	5	day	product X product Y	2
Action	avoid	avoid	avoid	suggest	avoid

The Arden Syntax [2] has been proposed as a pre-standard for the description of the medical knowledge in terms of medical logic modules. It receives a growing interest in the world of medical informatics and has already been studied in the context of pharmacological knowledge representation [3]; it is almost a de facto standard for medical knowledge based systems. We consequently compared our object oriented representation with the Arden syntax, which appears to be a conceptual subset of the MLM. In the maintenance section of MLM we are missing information dealing with system maintenance, directly related with implementation. The library section is totally missing except for the item 'purpose' which can be filled in OPADE by a string like 'satisfy a logical rule'; this section is needed for maintenance of the information. Finally the most important section of the MLM, the knowledge section, can totally be derived from the PP, but the structure of the 'logic' item is more constrained in OPADE by the allowed combinations contained in prescription features. There is consequently no problem to translate the OPADE within the Arden formalism whenever needed.

5. Discussion

In the design of OPADE, particular attention was paid to the integration of the system in clinical practice in an undisturbing way, while providing additional support through critiques, and suggestions.

Integration within medical practice means that the system must provide at least the existing level of working efficiency, while respecting local medical practice rules. Efficiency is taken care of by the fact that OPADE can directly be integrated with existing patient medical record and because it provides extended auto-completion allowing to automatically propose administration method and regimen of a patient prescription from the drug name and the indication. Respect of local medical practice rules is enforced by the evaluation within OPADE of the last category of PPs, the policy constraints, and more particularly the guidelines specified by the local and even national therapeutic committee. Following Example 6 provided in Section 2, if a physician does prescribe another treatment in case of hypertension he/she will be warned that this does not respect local guidelines. This may be considered as a positive feature by prescribers who want to follow local rules; it may also be considered as an intrusion in prescribing freedom. The later is a local infrastructure problem independent of the introduction of computers; OPADE helps to enforce local rules; if the prescriber does not like it, he/she can still disable the warning component of OPADE.

We believe also that a system such as OPADE - if well accepted and actually used - can introduce a positive feed back loop in the prescribing process. Indeed if OPADE is actually used by all prescribers within a clinical institution, the output of the system can be studied to identify prescription patterns at the individual or institutional level.

These patterns can be further analysed by the local therapeutic committee and new Prescribing Principles can be derived to correct bad prescribing practice and/or to enforce adequate practice. Once introduced in the system knowledge base, these new principles will be the source of new types of suggestions or reminders. Several studies have showed that clinicians' attitudes are influenced by a critiquing system [4,5,6]; it is hoped that the evolving critiques generated by OPADE will directly influence the prescribing attitude of clinicians.

We do not claim that Prescribing Principles as described here will all fulfil their expectations; more work is needed to evaluate their representation relatively to work on the representation of protocols and guidelines, to further validate their content and to actually measure their impact. We nevertheless believe that they represent an important step toward structuration in drug prescribing guidelines.

7. Acknowledgments

The OPADE project is partially funded by the Advance Informatics in Medicine (AIM) initiative of the EEC under contract number A2027. It is a 360 man months project which will last for three years, starting January 1992. The OPADE consortium is composed by the following partners: BIM (B), ISI -Bari University (I), IS - City University London (UK), Eclimed -University Paris V (F), Setec Informatique (F), Swedis DC (Sw) and Psychology Dept. - Reading University (UK). ICRF (UK) has been subcontracted to install and evaluate the system in UK.

8. References

[1]   A. Venot, B. Kostrewski et al. Deliverable D1. Study of Computerized Drug Prescription Systems. Public report of the OPADE project. April 1992.

[2]   G, Hripcsak, PD. Clayton, A. Pryor, P Haug, O. Wigertz and J.Van de Lei. The Arden syntax for medical logic modules. Proceedings of the 14th SCAMC meeting. Washington DC, 1990, 200-204

[3]   HU Prokosch, S, Kamm, D.Wieczorek and J. Dudeck. Knowledge representation in Pharmacology. A possible aplication area for the Arden syntax Proceedings AMIA, 1992, 243-247

[4]   F. Lau, D. Vincent. Formalized Decision-Support for Cardiovascular Intensive Care. Proceedings of 16th annual SCAMC meeting, 442-447, 1992.

[5]   R.S. Evans, S.L. Pestonik, D.C. Classn, S. Bass, J. Burke. Prevention of Adverse Drug Events through Computerized Surveillance. Proceedings of 16th annual SCAMC meeting, 437-442, 1992.

[6]   D.M. Rind, C. Safran, R.S. Phillips et al. The Effect of Computer-Based Reminders on the Management of Hospitalized Patients with worsening Renal function. Proceedings of 15th annual SCAMC meeting, 28-32, 1991

Health Telematics for Clinical Guidelines and Protocols
C. Gordon and J.P. Christensen (Eds.)
IOS Press, 1995

Integrating guidelines and the clinical record: the role of semantically constrained terminologies

Andrzej Glowinski

Biomedical Informatics Unit, Imperial Cancer Research Fund Laboratories, Lincoln's Inn Fields, London

Abstract. The extent to which protocols and guidelines will be used depends critically on how well they are integrated with existing medical records and each other. Effective integration requires consistent information structures and content, but if the union between components becomes too intimate it may restrict interaction with other applications. Such isolation leads to operational inefficiencies and can be financially unattractive. Systematic representation methods for protocols address part of the problem but are hampered by the unsuitability of existing medical terminologies; the effort required for bespoke development is prohibitive. Unifying and generalising terminological functions in a single "Terminology Server" that can support both construction of systems and their operational use promises to reduce development effort whilst allowing individual designers considerable independence. However, significant theoretical and practical questions remain about how far the problems of communication can be mitigated by a generalised, use-independent terminological system.

1 Introduction

Providing the highest quality of care and making the best use of available resources have been a concern in medicine throughout its history; witness the traditional maxim of "first, do no harm" – a goal that seems increasingly difficult to achieve in the face of ever advancing powers and ranges of treatment, and, paradoxically, a greater understanding of the underlying processes of disease and the mechanism of drug action. The paradox may in part be illusory, stemming from increasing standards and scrutiny, but one consequence nevertheless is the greater attention being paid to what is being done and how, and whether an acceptable balance between results and cost is being achieved.

Guidelines and protocols would seem to have a considerable role to play in improving quality and maximising effectiveness in medical care [1]; for examples, see [2,3]. However, developing a good protocol involves more than collating sound evidence and gaining consensus, as anybody who has ever used one will be aware: irrespective of validity, it must also be well formulated, presented and pertinent to the case under consideration – and above all, be accessible. As the range of conditions and circumstances addressed by protocols increases the problems of remembering that one is applicable, finding it and interpreting general guidance in the context of the individual circumstances of the patient can spiral. The potential for conflicting interactions between the advice offered by overlapping guidelines can grow exponentially, and will undoubtedly develop into a serious issue once protocols start to become mandatory for medico-legal or reimbursement purposes.

Recent years have seen increasing use of computers in supporting various aspects of protocol management, ranging from data collection for research purposes to provision of advice, even about the design of protocols themselves [4]. Computerised systems for protocol management have formed an important focus in Medical Informatics research for some time [5,6,7] but have repeatedly run into problems that have limited their use. On one hand, technical difficulties of knowledge representation, limited scope and the management of uncertainty have proved harder to overcome than initially hoped, but probably more significant are barriers preventing integration into everyday medical practice. These encompass:–

- **organisational aspects**: the system does not fit in to the way people work, especially when part of a team
- **the user interface**: often *inappropriately* (**rather than badly**) **designed**
- **the nature and form of the advice provided**: professionals performing complex tasks have specific but often poorly articulated **information requirements**
- **integration with other information repositories**: advisory systems need a great deal of clinical information to work well, and protocols are more demanding than most in this respect. Double entry of data is time consuming, prone to error and usually shunned.

This paper explores the last of these issues, specifically looking at the integration of protocols and guidelines with each other and with medical record systems, both from the perspectives of design and development and use. In particular, problems associated with communicating clinical information between systems that store and use will be considered, and the idea that a "Terminology Server" can be used to provide greatly extended, unified facilities aimed at overcoming the barriers of restricted, incompatible subsets of medical language, perhaps with multilingual capabilities, will be examined.

1.1 A note about guidelines and protocols

Although many authors make no strict distinctions between "protocols" and "guidelines", tending to use the terms interchangeably, it is perhaps useful to consider differences that may have operational consequences. On one hand, *guidelines* may be seen as statements of desirable goals and the principles to be used to achieve those goals, as distinct from *protocols* which convey detailed instructions about the steps that should – even must – be followed [8]. Along quite a different axis lies the ranking of the authority and applicability of protocols and guidelines, as discussed by Eddy [9]. The precision and force of instructions influence the quality and completeness of the clinical data that has to be available, and often the detail in the records that need to be kept – the difference between a chemotherapy protocol in oncological treatment and guidelines for the use of a simple drug regimen (as presented in many formularies) illustrate this well. For brevity, I will use the term *protocol system* here to refer to the whole spectrum of guideline and protocol management systems.

2 The problem of clinical data

Making clinical decisions well is an information-intensive activity; indeed, the quality and quantity of information available may even outweigh the influence of the decision making method used in some circumstances [10]. Omission of essential data about a case can introduce considerable biases or errors [11,12], so facilities for compiling a complete record are usually given prominence in the design of any system that depends on information about the patient. As previously mentioned, this can result in the system failing to gain acceptance not because of inadequacies in measurable performance but as a result of the demanding, machine-dominated style of interface this tends to lead to (for example, see [13]). Integrating the protocol system with an existing electronic patient record is an attractive means for reducing or eliminating data entry and improving data integrity, but is hampered because most clinical records are currently paper-based – a computerised protocol system has little chance of direct access to the data it needs.

Electronic clinical records (referred to in many ways – often as *electronic patient records*, or EPRs), like protocol systems, have been studied for some time, but many recent initiatives have contributed to much increased activity in both the storage and communication of patient data and in associated areas such as terminology and classification. For example, there are the collaborations under the auspices of the EC *Advanced Informatics in Medicine Program* (AIM), the work of the Clinical Patient Record Institute (CPRI) in the US, and many individual projects in other countries.

2.1 The relationship between protocols and records

Before looking at the requirements for passing relevant information between a protocol system and a clinical record and the methods available to support good communication it is worth examining the relationship between the systems themselves. These may be divided into three interrelated levels:–

- physical
- conceptual
- contextual

The remainder of this paper analyses some of the characteristics of concept representation from the perspective each of these levels, and the way these features affect the interaction of records and protocols. It goes on to examine the approaches that are currently being studied in an attempt to overcome some of the difficulties, and discusses their merits and several issues that remain outstanding.

3 The physical level – coupling clinical records and applications

The relationship between protocol systems (indeed, generally any medical decision support system) and the clinical record may be categorised as integrated, closely-coupled or loosely-coupled (see [14], chapter 10, for a general discussion of the integration of databases and knowledge bases).

Integrated systems. Most stand-alone medical advisory systems incorporate a bespoke, specific clinical record designed to hold only the data needed by the advice mechanism itself; there is usually little possibility of using (sometimes even accessing) patient data separately for any other purpose. The system is designed and implemented as a singular whole: many of the medical expert systems developed over the last 15 years come into this category. As pure clinical records such designs fall far short of what would be expected in a modern EPR both in terms of functionality and architecture. Although a system of this type may be adaptable to another problem or protocol, the re-engineering effort required to do this may be akin to starting from scratch. The most significant factors here are lack of separation of the components; the embedding of many functions that would need to be altered; and the specificity of (and implicit contexts within) the clinical terminology being used.

Tightly-coupled designs distinguish the record keeping and decision support sub-components and introduce a degree of functional independence to the implementation. These have become more common recently, especially where the focus of research has been on developing a system that can manage a variety of protocols (e.g. [15]). The clinical record is still dedicated to the protocol system, especially from the perspectives of content and structure, with specific semantic constraints often built into the implementation (usually implicitly at the level of the interface [16]). Data may be entered directly into the record but the requirements of the protocol determine what items are asked for, with the interface design driven exclusively by these considerations. The knowledge representation structure and elements recorded (frequently defined by means of a data dictionary) are tuned specifically to the needs of the decisions being made, so that it may even be impossible to record information about the patient that is clinically significant but irrelevant to the active protocol.

Although this arrangement may appear very restrictive, if well designed it can be extended to cope with a range of protocols (although usually of the same type – see the discussion of PROTÉGÉ [6]). However, if too many implicit assumptions about the knowledge structures and contents are present in the conceptual schema and information is excessively compiled into the implementation, it may prove very difficult to extend such a system because of semantic uncertainty or conflicts (this aspect is discussed further below). The scope for adaptation, however, is usually much greater than for an integrated system because of the separation of elements, and in a well-conceived application may make considerable use of the advantages that stem from having a clinical record structure and vocabulary that are wholly under control of the designer.

Loose coupling combines entirely separate information-using and clinical record elements, with the record in theory being available to all of the client applications that need clinical data. The components can be independently designed and implemented, an arrangement that should free the developer of the burden of having to build both application and data management system. Furthermore, an open design can allow sharing of common elements between systems, either in the form of passive libraries or active servers – using an existing terminological coding or classification scheme is an obvious choice here, and there is much experience of doing this especially in manual systems. The advent of client-server architectures has increased interest in such arrangements, and the level of investment required to build a comprehensive EPR suggests that they really do need to be multi-purpose to justify their development, with the capacity to supply information to as many different client applications as possible.

Lower costs of storage media and computational power are a prerequisite for large, distributed systems, but several other factors are even more important in moving towards a scenario that looks increasingly attractive and is apparently attainable. Development may be much more difficult in practice than may appear at first sight, with perhaps the most important factor being the need for effective transfer of highly complex information between components. Despite these caveats, the current trend appears to favour separate development of electronic medical records [17,18], often with no specific information-using application in mind.

4 The conceptual level – data models and information content

In the past, electronic patient records have been more concerned either with administrative information or data collection for aggregation – morbidity and mortality statistics, research, audit and financial purposes – than with individual patient care. The emphasis on grouping patients into sub-populations inevitably leads to simplified data models which concentrate on the uniform features of different patients and quite intentionally suppress certain elements of diversity. The conceptual schema of a record designed for this purpose is thus usually based on a highly selected subset of concepts and data types, with its structure specifically reflecting the aggregation of information demanded by this kind of application. Much that would be useful in different circumstances, particularly direct medical care with its ill-characterised and diverse information requirements, is thereby omitted or extremely difficult to represent within the confines of the schema.

It has been argued that an electronic patient record should be capable or representing all the clinically significant information found in paper records, even speculative notes and opinions, for it to be truly useful in everyday clinical work [19]. Two features that strongly distinguish an electronic record from its paper-based counterpart are its predetermined structure and regularity – the more methodical and ordered it is the greater the scope for useful manipulation of the data held. Fundamental prerequisites for systematic organisation include uniformity and predictability of the data held in the record; more accurately, the concepts represented and the relationships between them (the ontology of the domain) need to be formally and explicitly defined. Conventionally, this has in part been managed through the imposition of terminological coding and classification systems; however, most existing schemes were devised for epidemiological measurement [20] or reporting pathological findings [21] not for medical records, although more recent developments do attempt to address clinical issues (for instance [22]). Additionally, their ontologies are perhaps not as explicit nor regular as we might like, but for the restricted purposes they were intended for this does not usually matter.

Such schemes can usually be classified either as *enumerative*, defining all or most concepts in advance, or *combinatorial*, allowing essentially unrestricted conjunctions of elements. From the EPR viewpoint, the first approach can be unduly restrictive whilst the second can produce a combinatorial explosion of concepts, many of which are medically nonsensical [23]. For the medical record to function adequately as a support for applications that use the information it stores, the concept representation employed must possess a number of important properties:–

• it must be complete with respect to the application. All of the concepts that are required by the application must be capable of being represented. To estimate the degree of completeness both formal and empirical measures of completeness need to be employed, covering an exhaustive theoretical analysis of the properties of the scheme (is it *capable* of representing all of the concepts?) as well as performance in dealing with as large a number of examples as can be tested (*does* it contain all the concepts?).

• correctness must be demonstrable. The representation must not allow the existence or generation of computational ambiguity or medically nonsensical concepts (this is distinct from the representation of uncertainty, which must be allowed). Again, there are formal and empirical aspects of correctness to consider: *could* badly-formed concepts appear? *are* nonsensical items found?

• it should be consistent, both within itself ("intrinsic consistency") and with the applications that are linked to the record ("extrinsic consistency"). Information should be represented in the same way across the whole domain. Concepts must always be well formed in order to be effectively processed, interpreted, presented and exchanged; to achieve this, descriptions must be uniform across the whole spectrum of medicine dealt with by the applications and the EPR. This means avoiding common problems such as varying levels of detail (leading to incompatible granularity of description) and inconsistent selection of the features by which concepts are defined.

Significantly greater obstacles are encountered in satisfying these requirements in the domain of medicine than in many others due to the scale and complexity of the field. Constraints over what is "sensible" cannot be expressed solely at the abstracted, single level of the conceptual schema but need to extend to items normally regarded as part of the extension of the schema [16] (this aspect causes peculiar difficulties, and is returned to below).

4.1 Semantically constrained terminologies and terminology servers

The excessive restriction of expression attributable to pre-defined terminologies allied to the lack of control found in unrestrained compositional systems has prompted at least three avenues of exploration to find more promising alternatives. Many serious difficulties, not least on account of the scale of the task, have meant that the work has been slow, and important questions remain about the ultimate barriers to development: some of the most interesting, as well as practical, relate to the balance between expressivity and computational tractability which has been the subject of long-standing theoretical debate [24,25].

Enumerative schemes have been enhanced by the introduction of qualifiers, extending the range of variations of concepts that can be represented. For example, diseases can be graded according to severity. Although this approach can be affected by problems of controlling what is sensible – unless the groupings of concepts are homogeneous inconsistencies and exceptions become unacceptably frequent – it may well serve to extend established classifications without the need to abandon them wholesale. However, we await evaluations of the scope and effectiveness of these extensions.

Secondly, efforts are under way to control the concepts that can be produced by combinatorial systems by superimposing restrictive schemas or semantic constraints. Like the enumerative schemes, adding a set of secondary constructs is hampered by the structure that already exists; there may, for example, be too flat a classification to allow any but the broadest of groupings, and this is made more difficult by the inconsistencies that occur. However, such inconsistencies may have been unimportant at the time the scheme originated, and may only become apparent when viewed from the perspective of controlling interactions between elements. Two options are available: either to alter the structure to allow more accessible groupings, or produce a myriad of fine detail to achieve the desired level of control.

The third approach is to build an entirely new system, based on principles designed to cope with all of the requirements of scale, complexity, varying granularity and expressivity whilst affording sufficient control for the system to be usable. An example of this is the work undertaken in the GALEN project of the AIM Program [26]. This seeks to build a representational methodology based around a semantically constrained compositional system whose properties are well defined, formally specified and implemented in a representational language that provides all of the computational facilities needed to support practical applications [27,16].

The GALEN representation mixes specialisation of concepts by addition of semantically controlled attributes and values with asserted class membership and inheritance of properties (it is recognised that it is impossible in practice to describe *all* concepts as systematic derivatives of more general items). The system is generative (or deductive), allowing the intensional representation of a very large number of concepts all of which are guaranteed to be well formed and medically sensible because of the constraints applied. In addition, each will be correctly classified along all possible axes instead of just one or a small number as is the usual case.

There are features that – superficially at least – indicate a degree of convergence among these three approaches. All tend to be more concerned with concepts rather than terms; they deal with concepts that can be refined in some way, with control exerted over the nature of the refinement; all involve information that is too complex to store in the same way as conventional codes and classifications or manipulate by hand. Indeed, the computational power required to manage a fully featured semantically constrained compositional system is significant, but intermittently required. The approach adopted in GALEN is to centralise the terminological reasoning into a server: this extends the idea of decoupling application components and maximises the use of intermittently required resources. It also fits well with the development of client-server architectures and high-bandwidth communications, technologies which are now reaching maturity.

Such a "Terminology Server" would provide a range of services to any client that needed them, on demand, dealing with both definitional and classificatory aspects of the terminology. For instance:–

1   "what can I say about a concept?" or "how can I describe or refine this concept?"
2   "is this a legal, well-formed concept?"
3   "what sort of category does this concept fall into?"
4   "how does this concept relate to an existing classification or coding scheme?"
5   "are these two concepts, which happen to be differently named, the same or related?"

Question 1 might be asked when designing a building a patient record system, or creating a user interface that allows a user the facility to describe an item in as much detail as is desired (this can be done dynamically, as in the Pen&Pad system [28]). Question 2 is almost universal – any system that is concerned with maintaining integrity of data demands that all the items it contains are well-formed, but ensuring that (or even determining whether) this is the case can be very hard. Question 3 provides a basic classificatory mechanism; as mentioned above, the GALEN inference engine is heavily dependent on this. Question 4 extends this by mapping concepts onto existing coding and classification schemes, a process that may be more complex than appears at first sight because of the implicit information that most of these use to define their contexts.

4.2   Terminological matching for protocol and record integration

The last question, however, is perhaps the most interesting from the point of view of the designer trying to integrate a medical record and a protocol system, as it addresses the problem of matching fine-grained patient data to the more general principles as laid out in the protocol. This form of abstraction has long been discussed as part of the process of reasoning [29], but still causes innumerable problems – the patient data and the instructions of the protocol are presented at totally different levels of detail, and perhaps even using quite distinct nomenclatures. Here we have a proposal to generalise and formalise at least the terminological element. By using grounded compositional descriptions (along with explicitly asserted "kind of" statements) which may be quite separate from the labels used for concepts, matches can be found much more easily. This certainly promises a way of coping with the sort of question that is frequently met in practice, for example, does *"severe, persistent but fluctuating discomfort in the fifth left metacarpophalangeal joint"* in the patient record correspond to *"small joint symptoms"* in the protocol? Rather than rely on the knowledge engineer having to cover every such example and variation the Terminology Server should be able to cope with an infinite range of specialisations of *"small joint symptoms"*, so long as each is "medically sensible" (i.e. legally allowed by the constraints within the system).

4.3 Terminological matching for protocol and record design

Using a Terminology Server to integrate records and protocols at run time will overcome significant problems, but of greater potential is its use during design and implementation. In this respect, its function is similar to that of a conventional coding or classification system, but with much greater power: the engineer can be certain that any protocol system built with the help of a Server will be compatible with any EPR that uses the same Server, hence does not need to worry about classificatory matches. The implementers of an EPR can guarantee that the system will be terminologically compatible with any application that uses data stored in the record, so long as it has been designed using the Server – all terminological reasoning will be taken care of outside the application. In addition, the software can perform some of the very time consuming and intricate (even impossible) checks that are needed to detect interference between protocols, where the same topic is covered but the overlap is hidden by the use of dissimilar names. This is a growing concern amongst protocol developers, and has contributed to a noticeable slowing down of the rate of appearance of protocol "series" which aim to cover a wide range of common conditions.

5 Context and communication

The emergence of the notion of use-independent EPRs has necessitated a movement towards use-independent terminologies to support both representation of information and its communication. The extended terminologies that are now appearing all incorporate (to varying extents) the notion of a universal *canonical form* by which a concept may be represented, quite distinct from the "visible" labels attached to it [30].

There are, however, important issues that must be addressed before we can be certain that the claims made about this approach can be justified in full.

• Can such a universal, use-independent scheme actually support communication between applications (particularly records and reasoning mechanisms) without taking into account the context of communication?

• Can all of the necessary constructs be provided, or will there be a need for elements that make unacceptable computational demands?

• Are we in a position to manage the scale and complexity of an adequate Terminology Server, especially in the face of constantly changing medical knowledge and perspectives?

5.1 Context

Communication between applications involves more than sending the name of a concept, however richly structured and defined; the context within which the exchange of information takes place, the task being performed and the nature of the question being asked can all affect which aspects are important and which irrelevant. But the problem is that deciding which attributes are relevant depends almost entirely upon the task and the case under consideration: there will be many different, overlapping but coherent sets of attributes for any item [31], but which is the "right" one? This starts to become uncomfortably close to the system of "possible worlds" found in modal logics, and implies that severe complications could arise. The problem lies in the need for "semantic equivalence" – the information transferred has the same meaning to the two applications – and the difficulty in defining and ensuring such equivalence. Although the information transferred from a medical record may be superficially compatible with the client application, the absence of contextual specification may result in misinterpretation. For example, as qualifiers of uncertainty (confirmation, suspicion, absence, etc.) and intentions and plans are recorded in more detail simply passing the subject (symptom, diagnosis or treatment) can be misleading.

It is certainly feasible to imagine a concept representation system that copes well with a single application or a small set of very similar applications, but there is no evidence that complex systems, dealing with multiple, dissimilar tasks which use overlapping parts of the medical record can be supported by a terminology that has been designed pre-hoc without specific reference to its use.

5.2 Expressivity

Even if it is taken for granted that the problem of context can be overcome, the fact remains that each clinical situation is ultimately unique, and every question is couched in different terms – can unambiguous differentiation be achieved simply by selection of the appropriate attribute set? Allowing only stereotyped and restricted questions or an impoverished set of concept descriptions may allow the system to work, but does this reduce expressivity to an unusable degree? An alternative is to extend the quantity of information included in the description of a concept (adding to the set of available attributes) so that the context if explicitly included. Two factors come into play if this is done: the attributes start to become more assertional, which causes adverse effects on decidability and computational behaviour [32], and the size and complexity of each concept rise swiftly (even exponentially) as more facets are included [16], and can eventually become unmanageable.

5.3 Scale and complexity

Despite theoretical advances in managing the scale and complexity of medical records and terminological services, severe practical problems associated with building and maintaining such systems remain. In general, growth of complexity (and the knowledge acquisition effort required) is exponentially related to size; this is compounded when multiple client applications with potentially conflicting requirements and contexts are considered. The problem of managing interference between these requirements (which is related to issues of interoperability in databases, and may eventually manifest itself as difficulty in maintaining the integrity of the record) requires additional techniques above the constraint systems described above.   Software tools that provide model-based authoring and evaluation facilities are needed as the tasks involved are too complex to be carried out manually [33]. There is usually a wealth of relevant information in the ontology defined in the conceptual schemas of the tasks and the record, and the more abstract levels of the terminology, but the relationship of this to the tasks of editing and checking the contents is missing.   Most research and development projects have been concerned with building relatively small prototypes that support only one or two activities in a selected sub-domain of medicine – their purpose is usually to demonstrate the feasibility of the representational scheme and terminological services; issues of completeness, global correctness and extrinsic consistency especially tend to receive little attention because they do not impinge on the function when the application is small and the impact of complexity has not really been felt.

6 Discussion

Given that pressures for clinicians to use a variety of protocols are undoubtedly going to increase for various reasons (quality of care and cost containment amongst them), what are the implications for developments in medical informatics?

Client-server architectures have much to commend them and are rapidly gaining ground in the medical arena, but in comparison with traditional administrative and financial systems the great breadth and complexity of clinical information creates results in a larger number of serious problems.   Perhaps most important, however, is the variety of clinical tasks that the information has to support – even applying a protocol involves numerous separate activities with distinct but overlapping information requirements.   These factors combine to produce a mixture of demands that appear irreconcilable.

However, several promising approaches have emerged that may go some way to breaking through the chaos.   Exerting close control and imposing standards as widely as possible has always been effective, but the demands of new applications mean that traditional manual terminologies and classifications are inadequate; the new techniques make use of computational facilities, and fit well with the emerging client-server separation.   Considerable enthusiasm and ambitious claims have been made for these approaches, but serious questions remain about what will happen when the move from restricted prototypes to large demonstrators and real-time systems is made.

Long experience from a range of disciplines suggests that communication of information in open environments which allow many different and competing interpretations to be placed on the information that is stored and manipulated soon runs into severe problems of context and meaning.   Completely unrestricted access to the patient record by any application can lead to unpredictable results.   Ensuring that messages are semantically equivalent in these circumstances, anticipating that the Terminology Server will resolve all of the problems, will encounter difficulties that may prove insurmountable.   Indeed, the hope that a single structured clinical record can be general enough to be coupled to *any* conceivable client is probably unrealistic.

7 Conclusions

Despite these caveats, it seems that the principle of centralisation of terminological and similar reasoning services along with unification of representations where appropriate does offer considerable advantages, not least to the developer who can ignore some of the time consuming activities associated with terminology and communications. For any system to be worthwhile, however, it needs to be fully functional across all of the areas that it seeks to address, be accepted by the communities that it seeks to serve, and provide guarantees of quality, longevity, and compatibility with whatever already exists. The consequences of these considerations are far-reaching and encompass organisational as well as technical issues, but must be addressed for progress to be made. Work has progressed well in recent years, but much remains to be done, and significant shifts of emphasis and even direction are required if the results are to be practically usable. As in many areas of informatics, evaluation and quantification of performance, effort and cost are required, and objective comparisons between methods and the consequences of restricting or extending the scope of a service are sorely needed.

References

[1] Grimshaw J M, Russell I T (1993) Effect Of Clinical Guidelines On Medical-practice - A Systematic Review Of Rigorous Evaluations Lancet 342 1317-1322

[2] Timothy A R, Brewin T, Chamberlain J et al (1988) Cost versus benefit in non-surgical management of patients with cancer BMJ 297 471-472

[3] Karjalainen S, Paula I (1989) Do treatment protocols improve end results? A study of survival of patients with multiple myeloma in Finland BMJ 299 1069-1072

[4] Wyatt J C, Altman D G, Heathfield H A, Pantin C F A (1994) Development of Design-a-Trial, a knowledge-based critiqueing system for authors of clinical trial protocols Computer Methods and Programs in Biomedicine 43 283-291

[5] Shortliffe E H, Scott A C, Bischoff B, et al (1984) Oncocin: an expert system for oncology protocol management In: Rule based expert systems: the MYCIN experiments of the Stanford Heuristic Programming Project ed. Buchanan B, Shortliffe E H. Addison-Wesley, Reading MA, 653-668

[6] Musen M A, Fagan L M, Combs D M, Shortliffe E H (1987) Use of a domain model to drive an interactive knowledge-editor International Journal of Man-Machine Studies 26 105-121

[7] Zanstra P E Computerised assessment with primary care guidelines in the Netherlands This volume

[8] Jenkins D (1991) Investigations: how to get from guidelines to protocols BMJ 303 323-324

[9] Eddy D M (1990) Practice policies - guidelines for methods JAMA 263 1839-1841

[10] O'Neil M J, Glowinski A J (1990) Evaluating and validating very large knowledge-based systems Medical Informatics 15 237-252

[11] Dawes RM, Corrigan B (1974) Linear Models in Decision Making Psychological Bulletin 81 95-106

[12] Heckerling PS, Elstein AS, Terzian CG, Kushner MS (1991) The effect of incomplete knowledge on the diagnoses of a computer consultant system Medical Informatics 16 363-370

[13] Lindberg D A B, Humphreys B L (1990) The UMLS knowledge sources:tools for building better user interfaces Proceedings of the 14th Annual Symposium on Computer Applications in Medical Care (SCAMC) IEEE New York 121-125

[14] Garadani G, Valduriez P (1989) Relational database and knowledge bases Addison Wesley 315-377

[15] Gordon C, Herbert S I, Jackson-Smale A, Renaud-Salis J-L (1993) Care protocols and healthcare informatics Technology and informatics 10 - Artificial Intelligence in Medicine, IOS Press 289-309

[16] Goble C A, Glowinski A J, Jeffery K G (1993) Semantic constraints in a medical information system Proceedings of BNCOD11 Lecture Notes in Computer Science. Springer Verlag 696 40-57

[17] Rector AL, Nowlan WA, Kay S, Goble CA, Howkins TJ (1992) A Framework for Modelling the Electronic Medical Record Methods of Information in Medicine 32, 109-119

[18] Dick R (1991) The computer-based patient record : an essential technology for health care Washington, D.C. : National Academy Press

[19] Rector A L, Nowlan W A, Kay S (1991) Foundations for an electronic medical record Methods of Information in Medicine 30 179-186

[20] World Health Organisation, Geneva. International Classification of Diseases (ICD)

[21] College of American Pathologists. Systematized Nomenclature Of Medicine (SNOMED International). Skokie, Illinois, USA: College of American Pathologists, 1993.

[22] Read Clinical Classification Developers and User Guides. Computer Aided Medical Systems Limited (CAMS), Loughborough, UK.

[23] Goble C A, Glowinski A J, Nowlan W A, Rector A L (1993) A descriptive semantic formalism for medicine Proceedings of the IEEE Ninth International Conference on Data Engineering, Vienna. IEEE Computer Society Press 624-632

[24] Levesque H J, Brachman R J (1985) A fundamental tradeoff in knowledge representation and reasoning. Readings in Knowledge Representation ed. Brachman R J, Levesque H J. Morgan Kaufmann, Los Altos, California 412-429

[25] Doyle J, Patil R S (1991) Two theses of knowledge representation Artificial Intelligence 48 261-297

[26] Rector A L, Nowlan W A, Glowinski A J (1993) Goals for concept representation in the GALEN project Proc. 17th SCAMC. McGraw-Hill: Washington DC 414-418

[27] Rector A L, Nowlan W A, Glowinski A J, et al (1993) GALEN Deliverable 6: The Master Notation The GALEN Consortium for the European Commission AIM Programme (Available from the Medical Informatics Group, University of Manchester).

[28] Rector A L, Goble C A, Horan B, et al (1990) Shedding light on patients' problems: integrating knowledge based systems into medical practice ECAI 90 531-534

[29] Clancey W J (1985) Heuristic Classification Artificial Intelligence 27 289-350

[30] Evans DA, Cimino J, Hersch WR et al (1994) Position statement: towards a medical concept representation language J. Am. Medical Informatics Assoc. 1 207-217

[31] Tversky A (1977) Features of similarity Psychological Review 84 327-352

[32] Brachman RJ, Levesque HJ (1984) The tractability of subsumption in frame-based description languages AAAI-84 34-37.

[33] Glowinski A J, Coiera E W, O'Neil M J (1991) The role of domain models in maintaining consistency of large medical knowledge bases Proceedings of the Third AIME Lecture Notes in Medical Informatics 44 72-81

Health Telematics for Clinical Guidelines and Protocols
C. Gordon and J.P. Christensen (Eds.)
IOS Press, 1995

Framework for quality assessment of knowledge*)

J. Brender[a], J. Talmon[b], P. McNair[c]

[a]Medical Informatics Laboratory ApS, Stengaards Allé 33d, DK-2800 Lyngby, Denmark.
[b]University of Limburg, Dept. of Medical Informatics, P.O.Box 616, 6200 MD
Maastricht, The Netherlands.
[c]Hvidovre Hospital, Dept. of Clinical Chemistry 339, DK-2650 Hvidovre, Denmark.

Abstract. One of the key issues in the development (and subsequent application) of medical knowledge - be it in terms of a KBS or otherwise - is the assessment of its quality. We present a framework for how to manage and make measurable the quality of the semantic as well as pragmatic aspects of the knowledge embedded in classification models during the development of such models.

1 Introduction

The KAVAS and KAVAS-2[1] AIM Projects have developed a framework for the assessment of quality of (executable) classification models [Brender et al. 1990a, 1990b]. It has the purpose of managing and making measurable the quality of classification models in the semantic sense and in relation with its usefulness in application. Although the framework was designed for the assessment of Knowledge-Based Systems in medicine it is generally applicable.

The emphasis in this contribution will be on the pragmatic issues of quality assessment during the development of classification models.

1.1 The KAVAS approach for development of classification models

KAVAS-2's main objective is to develop a toolbox, named KAVIAR ("Knowledge Acquisition, VIsualisation Assessment and Refinement"), to be used by medical experts for developing and assessing domain knowledge. Innovative elements of KAVIAR are the following key functionalities [Brender et al. 1993a]: 1) built-in quality assessment of semantic aspects of knowledge [Brender et al. 1993b], 2) features for controlling the machine learning process in order to make it focus on the desired qualities, a process called Conditioning [Talmon et al. 1991, McNair et al. 1993], and 3) coupling of machine learning techniques with knowledge elicitation techniques thereby enabling the support of the user in varying clinical situations where different data and knowledge sources are available.

---

*) Reprinted from "Advances in Knowledge Organisation, vol.4 (1994): Knowledge Organization and Quality Management. Proceedings of the Third International ISKO Conference, Copenhagen June 1994. INDEKS Verlag:Frankfurt/Main." with permission from INDEKS Verlag.

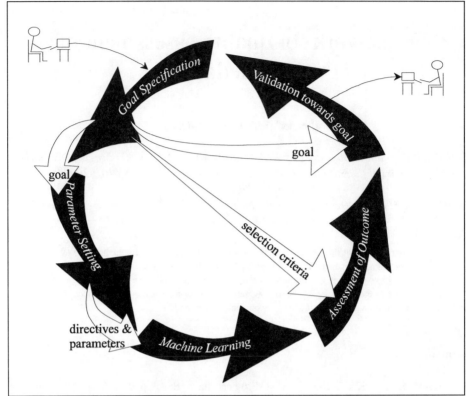

Figure 1: KAVIAR's learning cycle for the development of classification models.

The process of using KAVIAR compares to an iterative learning process:

1)   Goal definition, i.e. the formulation of the medical problem approached and elicitation of conditioning information.

2)   Selection (and parameter setting) of appropriate tools and techniques to be applied on the basis of among others the medical problem focused on and the conditioning information.

3)   Application of the selected tool(s).

4)   Measuring and exploring the characteristics and quality of the domain models.

5)   Validation of the domain models against the defined goals, leading to either a new learning iteration or to an implicit or explicit acknowledgement or rejection of the outcome.

These five operational steps correspond to the conceptual steps for tasks' accomplishment in general: goal clarification, selection of means, carrying out the task, and assessment of task, see Figure 1.

Presently, three machine learning techniques are implemented in KAVIAR: 1) an induction tool providing decision trees (i.e. protocols), 2) a neural network tool for creating feed-forward networks, trained by the back-propagation mechanism, and 3) a density inference algorithm which provides a probabilistic estimate of which class(es) in a given clinical database the case at hand resembles most. Further, tools are implemented for a) definition and formalisation of concepts e.g. by capturing them from a text, b) representation of (semantic) relations between concepts (Conceptual Graph tool), and c) representation of procedural knowledge (State-Transition-Diagram tool), - supporting the modelling of knowledge of various epistemological types (causal, goal-oriented, dynamic, context and basic biomedical knowledge). The latter tools have a dual purpose: to enable the user in formulating his own knowledge as a means for validation of the classification models, and to support the other tools (conditioning tools, the machine learning tools and the quality assessment tool) in circumscribing the clinical problem and needs.

KAVIAR may be seen as a Decision Support System for the development of clinical protocols. The learning process can be managed at any level of automation. The most automated being the one that builds models purely on the basis of the optimality criteria implemented in the tools; this is the approach taken in most implementations of induction algorithms. At the other extreme, support in data inspection is provided and full user control of all parameter settings for the involved tools is feasible. The induction tool has a manual mode, where the tool supports the user in each decision during the tree building process. All intermediate levels of human intervention between these extremes are feasible and supported by KAVIAR.

KAVAS's philosophy is to develop and validate classification models by means of several supplementary (and integrated) tools and techniques. Classification models based on machine learning techniques are by nature executable, but it is up to the user to implement them in clinical practice either as computer-based or paper-based classification models.

1.2 Quality Assessment during the development of clinical protocols

The purpose of the framework for quality assessment and its implementation in the KAVIAR tool is to make it an integrated part of the entire process of development of clinical protocols and other classification models, and to enable users to fully assess the resulting models. The overall approach is that of integrating development and evaluation to enable iterative refinement cycles leading to a satisfactory result. The user requirements (i.e. the conditioning information) as regards the required classification model are quality aspects like predictive values, coverage as well as ethical and economical constraints [McNair ct al. 1993]. They serve 1) as a basis for tool parameter settings and/or 2) in a multivariate criteria analysis as a basis for selection among numerous candidate classification models. Finally, they serve as means for the quality assessor functionality in providing the user with information on the degree of fulfilment of user requirements and on potential reasons for experienced deviations, see Figure 1.

It is clearly seen that the quality management with an active and explicit quality assurance is integrated in the entire set-up of the learning process in KAVIAR from the point of specification of goals and requirements to the final assessment of outcome.

2 The Quality Assessment Framework

Most of the traditional quality measures of semantic aspects of medical knowledge are confined to 2 class problems (like Predictive Values, Sensitivity and Specificity) and/or have the assumption that all cases are labelled. These assumptions are not always fulfilled and one often is confronted with multiclass problems. The framework has served not only as a design principle but also as a means for structuring the development of new and generalised metrics and measures.

The KAVAS Framework for quality assessment constitutes a high level semantic description of quality management. It is composed of a set of orthogonal perspectives [Brender et al. 1993b] containing several concepts. Only a subset of these perspectives and their concepts will be addressed here:

a) The Quality Concepts Perspective, providing a comprehensive view on various aspects of quality.

b) The Quality Management Perspective, structuring the activities of a process ensuring the fulfilment of quality needs.

c) The Metrology Perspective, covering concepts in measurement of quality.

d) The Perception Perspective dealing with conceptual viewpoints on the quality concepts.

2.1 Quality Concepts Perspective

A literature study revealed that many quality concepts are defined at a measurement level, while only a few are defined at a conceptual level. Moreover, when a quality concept embraces only one measure this is often mistaken as identical with the concept itself. For instance, "correctness" is the term used everywhere in the literature when dealing with quality of KBS application. However, the literature does not discriminate between the quality concept itself and the measures (percentage of correct classifications) which characterise it and which are concepts in themselves.

In [Brender et al. 1990 a and b] we defined a preliminary minimum set of meta-knowledge (quality) concepts by generalisation and harmonization of quality concepts used in various domains. The notion of meta-knowledge stems from the perspective of quality of knowledge as knowledge-about-knowledge ("meta-X" is defined as "X about X" [Aiello et al.1986]) [2] .

The quality concepts were acquired by review of the literature in four medical domains, computer science and medical informatics and subsequently generalised and abstracted. The concepts identified are connected on the one hand to quality assurance of semantics of the knowledge-base and properties of the KB(S). On the other hand, they provide the basis for the assessment of possible consequences of application of the KB(S) in a given environment. For some of these concepts, one can define metrics and measures which can be obtained by examination of the KB(S) or by exercising the KB(S) with one or more sets of cases, while other measures require human intervention to achieve their measurement.

Examples of the former type of quality concepts are e.g. correctness, coverage, robustness, model complexity, problem solving strength, and goodness of fit, and examples of the latter are e.g. usefulness and reliability.

2.2 The Quality Management Perspective

Quality Management (QM) is the act of dealing with quality in a goal oriented and structured way. Within QM there are three concepts constituting a layered operational structure: quality assurance (QA), quality control (QC) and quality inspection (QI).

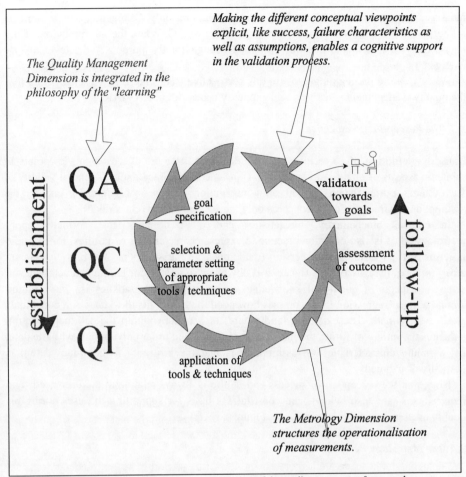

Figure 2: The KAVIAR learning cycle in view of the quality assessment framework.

From the ISO definition[3] it may be concluded that implementation of a quality policy implies that a goal and an approach/strategy for the goal's accomplishment have to be established; the goal serving as a frame of reference for further activities. This process is called QA. QA is concerned with strategic issues (objectives, premises) and planning activities (e.g. selection of methods) to ensure the desired level of quality.

The operationalisation of QA on the concrete problem case is the QC; the pragmatic set-up of relevant work processes is the QI. QC is concerned with combining and setting up the selected methods on the concrete problem case to meet the goal and fulfil other strategic decisions. QI is concerned with practical aspects in the measurement of individual measures. These three aspects function in a conceptual hierarchy of increasing abstraction from QI to QC and further on to QA. Each of these levels are operationally linked to the other levels.

The above description highlights the establishment part of QM. However, there is implicitly also a follow-up part of the QA, QC and QI in the ISO definitions to maintain the fulfilment of the quality policy: the most simple quality assessment constitutes the measurement part of the QI alone, i.e. providing measures only. QI together with a frame of reference for the quality measures lead to the level of QC. When the interpretation of the measures is related to the question of "good enough for the purpose?" the level of QA emerges.

When viewing the learning cycle in this perspective (see Figure 2) it is easily seen that the quality management is actively and explicitly dealt with in KAVIAR.

2.3 The Perception Perspective

From the definition of correctness[4] it is clear that there are at least two viewpoints in semantic aspects of quality of knowledge: i) the success characteristics ("general validity of the system's output when applied on a population of cases of interest"), and ii) the assumptions characteristic ("it concerns only those cases that are classified").

In clinical biochemistry, biostatistics and other domains that formally apply metrology[5], it is also common practice to express characteristics of failures, for example in terms of the measures of dispersion (randomness in measurement) and bias (systematic error) (see e.g. [Magid 1992]). Hence, it is obvious also to look for failure characteristics in semantic aspects of quality of knowledge. An example from statistics is: the variation around a linear regression line expresses how good the model fits the data, i.e. it constitutes a success estimate. The existence (and nature) of a pattern within the residual variation indicates the failure of fitting the model chosen (e.g. a 2nd order polynomial) with the data, i.e. a failure characteristic. An assumption is that the error of an individual datum is normally distributed.

Note, that the perception of success and failure is always relative to the user needs and requirements (see also below), and constitutes a basis for supporting the user during his quality assessment of the outcome, see Figure 2.

2.4 The Metrology Perspective

The hierarchy within the concepts of measurement is methodology, methods, metrics and measures. A methodology comprises the global approach (goal definition and strategies) together with a consistent and coherent set of methods from which one may select and combine a subset to achieve the goal; a method is a formalized description (including theories, application range and assumptions) for accomplishing a task; a metric is a formalized procedure or technique for measuring a quality or characteristic, therein also its basic theoretical framework; and a measure is a named concept that may bear a value.

The methodology is related with the information need and serves as the context for fully interpreting the measures. Methods have assumptions and therefore add to the context for interpretation of measures. One methodology may have numerous alternative methods to be applied for a task, and one method may be applicable within numerous methodologies.

The idea is that for each of the quality concepts identified (defined preliminary in [Brender et al. 1990 a and b]) there shall exist a methodology for establishing and interpreting their value, by means of the methods, their operational formula (the metrics) and the measures to which they give a value.

Viewed in KAVIAR's perspective, the methodologies and methods are implicitly implemented in the quality assessment and the conditioning, while the metrics are the actual calculations to be performed. The measures within their context for interpretation are the pieces of information to visualize towards the user during the quality assessment (see Figure 2).

2.5 *Practical aspects in assessment of quality of knowledge*

From the above four sections it is clear how the mentioned perspectives within the quality assessment framework relate with the actual learning process in KAVIAR.

The user of KAVIAR normally operates with a learning database and one or more test databases, of which some may be derived artificially to assess e.g. the vulnerability towards added noise on the attribute values (the robustness quality concept). Application of the generated classification algorithms on these populations of cases provides a lot of information which may be further processed into the actual quality measures.

KAVAS-2 has experimented with metrics and measures for a number of quality estimates [Brender et al. 1994, Egmont-Petersen et al. 1994]. For instance, we have identified several quality measures for the quality concept correctness:

- overall conformance (concerned with all classes and cases), label respectively class conditional conformance (concerned with conformance of the labelling respectively the true class)
- overall and conditional Kappa conformance (conformance corrected for the proportion of outcome classifications that appear by chance)
- bias.

In medicine, it is often not equally important to distinguish class A from class B as it is to distinguish class B from class A. In a situation where the distinction shall be made between say normals and cancer cases it is important not to overlook a cancer and may be unimportant to include a (small) proportion of normals into a group of cancer candidates which anyway will be prone to further clinical examinations and selections before initiation of a treatment. This means that the information theoretic optimality is not the same as the ethical optimality. The user (clinician) will require a classification model that has a bias reflecting his clinical situation. Hence, even large biases may be desirable, and therefore, what is relevant as the frame of reference in the quality assessment of a model is the deviation from this user requirement. Hence, what constitutes the success and the failure characteristics in a given quality assessment session entirely depends on the user requirements (the goal specification) for the classification models.

5 Conclusion

The major quality of the framework for quality assessment of knowledge is the structure which supports the development of quality measures. However, the framework has not only enabled the development of such quality measures. More important, it constitutes an integrated part of the design of the KAVIAR tool, supporting the user and enabling an active quality management in his development of classification models. As it stands now the framework constitutes a starting point for explicit quality management during the development of knowledge-based systems.

Note, that there is a distinction between quality assessment in the development phase and the application phase of a classification model. The former is population-oriented, while the latter is case-oriented. However, the framework may serve as a basis also for the development of metrics and measures in this respect.

Notes

[1]   KAVAS is an acronym for "Knowledge Acquisition, Visualization and Assessment System"

[2]   Meta-knowledge is "knowledge about knowledge", and as knowledge is a perception of causal relations and associations, meta-knowledge becomes "knowledge about causal relations and associations", which we interpret as "knowledge about qualities and characteristics of the perception of causal relations and associations". When expressed in an operational form, meta-knowledge may be defined as "knowledge about when, how, why and to what extent the knowledge can be applied and with what level of quality and confidence", i.e the concepts of meta-knowledge "bear" the values and the context for interpretation of quality of knowledge.

[3]   According to [ISO 8402, 1986] Quality Management is "that aspect of the overall management function that determines and implements the quality policy"; Quality Assurance is the "establishment and follow-up of strategies, including objectives, premises and methods applied to achieve the desired level of quality" (adapted from the ISO definition to achieve the same grammatical form from); Quality Control is the "establishment and follow-up of procedures, thereby operationalizing the strategies for a concrete case" (adapted from the ISO definition to achieve the same grammatical form; and Quality Inspection is the "establishment and measurement of individual quality measures" (ISO has no definition for quality inspection, but defines inspection as "activities such as measuring, examining, testing, gauging one or more characteristics of a product or service and comparing these with specified requirements to determine conformity".

[4]   Correctness is defined as "the general validity of the system's output when applied on a population of cases of interest"; correctness is meaningless, when (part of) input information is clinically inconsistent or when the knowledge is not applicable. Hence, it concerns only those cases that are classified."

[5]   Metrology is the science of measurement.

Acknowledgements

This work was partly funded by the Commission of the European Communities under the AIM Exploratory Action (KAVAS (A1021) Project) and the AIM Telematics in Health Care Program (KAVAS-2 (A2019) Project).

References

Aiello L.; Cecchi C.; Sartini D. (1986). Representation and Use of Metaknowledge. Proc IEEE 74(10), pp. 1304-1321

Brender J.; McNair P.; Raun H.; Nolan J.; Vingtoft, S. (1990a) Meta-knowledge as a Means for Quality Management in Knowledge-Based Systems. In: O'Moore R.R..; et al. (eds.): Lecture Notes in Medical Informatics 40, pp. 360-367

Brender J.; McNair P.; Raun H.; Nolan J.; Vingtoft S. (1990b). Meta-knowledge Concepts. Technical Report META-1.1 2nd ed., KAVAS (A1021) AIM Project, 34p.

Brender J.; Talmon J.; Nykänen P.; O'Moore R.; Drosos P.; McNair P. (1993a). KAVAS-2: Knowledge Acquisition Visualisation and Assessment System. In: Andreassen S.; Engelbrecht R.; Wyatt J. (eds.): Studies in Health Technology and Informatics: Artificial Intelligence in Medicine. Amsterdam:IOS Press. 10, pp. 417-420

Brender J.; Talmon J.; Egmont-Petersen M.; Schiøler T.; McNair P. (1993b). KAVAS's Framework for quality assessment of medical knowledge. In: Andreassen S.; Engelbrecht R.; Wyatt J. (eds.): Studies in

Health Technology and Informatics: Artificial Intelligence in Medicine. Amsterdam:IOS Press. 10, pp. 421-424

Brender J.; Talmon J.; McNair P. (1994). Measuring quality of medical knowledge. In: Proceedings of MIE'94, Lisbon 23-26th May 1994 (in press).

Egmont-Petersen M.; Talmon J.; Brender J.; McNair P. (1994). On the Quality of Neural Net Classifiers. Artificial Intelligence in Medicine (in press)

International Organization for Standardization (1986). Quality - Vocabulary. First edition - 1986-06-15 Ref. No. ISO 8402-1986 (E/F/R), 14p.

Magid E. (ed.) (1992). Some concepts and principles of clinical test evaluation. Classification, analytical performance, monitoring and clinical interpretation. Scand J Clin Lab Invest 52(suppl. 208), 132p.

McNair P.; Karthaus V.; Talmon J.; Thygesen H.; Schiøler T.; Brender J. (1993). KAVAS's Conditioning of the Induction Algorithm. In: Andreassen S.; Engelbrecht R.; Wyatt J. (eds.): Studies in Health Technology and Informatics: Artificial Intelligence in Medicine. Amsterdam:IOS Press. 10, pp. 425-428

Talmon, J.L.; Braspenning P.; Brender J.; McNair P. (1991). Machine Learning in data rich domains - Some experiences from the KAVAS project. In: Stefanelli M.; Hasman A.; Fieschi M.; Talmon J. (eds.): Lecture Notes in Medical Informatics 44, pp. 283-293

Select Bibliography

Compiled by Ian Purves
The Sowerby Unit for Primary Care Informatics, The Medical School,
University of Newcastle, Newcastle-on-Tyne NE2 4HH, UK

Abendroth TW, Greenes RA. A clinical algorithm processor: Enabling flow charts to organise a variety of physicians tasks. Proc Annu Symp Comput Appl Med Care 1989:983–984.

Abendroth TW, Greenes RA, Joyce EA. Investigations in the use of clinical algorithms to organise medical knowledge. Proc Annu Symp Comput Appl Med Care 1988:90–95.

Acute pain management guideline panel (Ed.). Acute pain management: Operative or medical procedures and trauma. (92-0032) (Clinical Practice Guideline.) Agency for Health Care Policy and Research Publications, Rockville, MD. 1992.

Anonymous. Guidelines for Doctors in the New World. Lancet 1992;339:1197–1198.

Audet AM, Greenfield S, Field M. Medical practice Guidelines: Current Activities and Future Directions. American College of Physicians 1990;113, No. 9.:709–714.

Bailey RD. Hypertension guidelines. Br Med J 1993;306:1337 (Letter).

Bainbridge M, Cowley C. Measuring health gain in patients: an integrated approach. In: HC92: Current perspectives in health care computing. (Ed: Richards,B) Br J Health Care Computing Books, Surrey. 1992. 32–38.

Barnett GO, Winickoff R, Dorsey JL, Morgan M, Lurie RS. Quality assurance through automated monitoring and concurrent feedback using computer-based medical information system. Medical Care 1978;16:962–970.

Barnett GO, Winickoff RN, Morgan MM, Zielstorff RD. A computer based monitoring system for follow-up of elevated blood pressure. Medical Care 1983;21:400–409.

Beaumont R. Care Pathways. In: Towards a Nursing Research Strategy for HTA. Centre for Health Services Research, Newcastle-Upon-Tyne. 1994. 1–13.

Beckers WPA, de Vries Robbe PF, Zanstra PE, Zwaard AM. Generic GP-Guidelines and Reasoning. 1993;4 May:1–10.

Berman L, Miller RA. Problem area formation as an element of computer aided diagnosis: a comparison of two strategies within quick medical reference (QMR). Methods Inf Med 1991;30(2):90–95.

Brook RH. Practice Guidelines and Practicing Medicine. Are They Compatible? JAMA 1989;262(21):3027–3030.

Brownridge G, Evans A, Fitter M, Platts M. An interactive computerised protocol for the management of hypertension: effects on the general practitioners clinical behaviour. J R Coll Gen Pract 1986;36:198–202.

Chambers CV, Balaban DJ, Carlson BL, Ungemack JA, Grasberger DM. Microcomputer generated reminders. Improving the compliance of primary care physicians with mammography screening guidelines. J Fam Pract 1989;3:273–280.

Charlton BG. Management of science. Lancet 1993;342:99–100.

Cohen DI, Littenberg B, Wetzel C, Neuhauser DB. Improving physician compliance with preventative medicine guidelines. Medical Care 1982;20:1040–1045.

Coleman RL. Promoting quality through managed care. American Journal of Medical Quality 1992;7(4):100–105.

Coste J, Delecoeuillerie G, Cohen de Lara A, Le Parc JM, Paolaggi JB. Clinical course and prognostic factors in acute low back pain: an inception cohort study in primary care practice. Br Med J 1994;308:577–581.

Coulter A, Bradlow J, Martin-Bates C, Agass M, Tulloch A. Outcome of general practitioner referrals to specialist outpatient clinics for back pain. Br J Gen Pract 1991;41(352):450–453.

Cousins SB, Frisse ME, Chen W, Mead CN. Stochastic simulation algorithms for query networks. Proc Annu Symp Comput Appl Med Care 1991:696–700.

Cowan JA, Heckerling PS, Parker JB. Effect of a fact sheet reminder on performance of the periodic health examination: a randomized controlled trial. Am J Prev Med 1992;8(2):104–109.

Davidson RA, Fletcher SW, Retchie S, Duh S. A nurse intiated reminder system for the periodic health examination: implementation and evaluation. Arch Intern Med 1984;144:2167–2170.

Delamothe T. Wanted: guidelines that doctors will follow. Implementation is the problem. Br Med J 1993;307:218 (Letter).

Deller Lorraine Spranzo, McDermott Susan, Alt-White Anna. Effects of Computerized Nurse Careplanning on Selected Health Care Effectiveness Measures. Proc Annu Symp Comput Appl Med Care 1992:38–42.

Detsky AS, Sackett DL. When was a "negative" clinical trial big enough ? Arch Intern Med 1985;145:709–712.

DiJerome L. The nursing case management computerised system: Meeting the challenge of health care delivery through technology. Computers in Nursing 1992;10(6):250–258.

Dolan JG, Bordley DR. Using the analytic hierarchy process (AHP) to develop and disseminate guidelines. QRB Qual Rev Bull 1992;18(12):440–447.

Durinck M, Coiera E. The role of knowledge based systems in clinical practice. In: Knowledge and Decisions in Health Telematics. (Eds: Barahona,P; Christensen,JP) IOS Press, Amsterdam. 1994. 199–203.

Eddy DM. Clinical decision making: from theory to practice. Designing a practice policy. Standards, guidelines, and options. JAMA 1990;263(22):3077,3081,3084.

Eddy DM. Clinical decision making: from theory to practice. Guidelines for policy statements: the explicit approach. JAMA 1990;263(16):2239–40,2243.

Eddy DM. Clinical decision making: from theory to practice. Practice policies - guidelines for methods. JAMA 1990;263(13):1839–1841.

Eddy DM. Clinical decision making: from theory to practice. Resolving conflicts in practice policies. JAMA 1990;264(3):389–391.

Eddy DM. Practice Policies - What are they ? JAMA 1990;263(6):877–880.

Eddy DM. Practice policies: where do they come from? JAMA 1990;263(9):1265, 1269, 1272.

Elliott CG. Computer-assisted quality assurance: development and performance of a respiratory care program. QRB Qual Rev Bull 1991;17(3):85–90.

Emslie CJ, Grimshaw J, Templeton A. Do clinical guidelines improve general practice management and referral of infertile couples? Br Med J 1993;306:1728–1731.

Evans AR, Wilkes ER, Absolon PJ, Denner TJ, Kaye G. An interactive computerised protocol for the management of hypertension. Methods Inf Med 1985;24:21–26.

Field MJ, Lohr KN (Eds.). Clinical practice guidelines: Directions for a new program. National Academy Press, Washington, DC. 1990.

Field MJ, Lohr KN (Eds.). Guidelines for Clinical Practice: From Development to Use. National Academic Press, Washington,DC. 1992.

Fink Arlene, Kosecoff Jacqueline, Chassin Mark, Brook Robert H. Consensus Methods: Characteristics and Guidelines for Use. Am J Public Health 1984;74, No. 9:979–983.

Franklin Rodney CG, Spiegelhalter David J, Macartney Fergus J, Bull Kate. Evaluation of a diagnostic algorithm for heart disease in neonates. Br Med J 1991;302:935–9:296–300.

Goldberg HI, Cummings MA, Steinberg EP, Ricci EM, Shannon T, Soumerai SB, Mittman BS, Eisenberg J, Heck DA, Kaplan S, et al. Deliberations on the dissemination of PORT products: translating research findings into improved patient outcomes. Med Care 1994;32(7, Suppl):JS90–J110.

Goodwin Donna R. Critical Pathways in Home Healthcare. JONA 1992;22(2):35–40.

Grampian Asthma Study of Integrated Care (GRASSIC). Effectiveness of routine self monitoring of peak flow in patients with asthma. Br Med J 1994;308:564–567.

Grampian Asthma Study of Integrated Care (GRASSIC). Integrated care for asthma: a clinical, social, and economic evaluation. Br Med J 1994;308:559–564.

Granneman T. Priority setting: A sensible approach to Medicaid policy? Inquiry 1991;28:300–305.

Greco PJ, Eisenberg JM. Changing physicians' practices. N Engl J Med 1993;329(17):1271–1273.

Green LW. How physicians can improve patients' participation and maintenance in self-care. West J Med 1987;147(3):346–349.

Green LW. Prevention and Health Education. Chap. 45. In: Public Health & Preventative Medicine. 13th ed. (Eds: Last,JM; Wallace,RB) Appleton & Lange, Norwalk, Connecticut. 1991. 787–802.

Greenes RA. "Desktop Knowledge": A new focus for medical education and decision support. Methods Inf Med 1989;28:332–339.

Greenfield S, Lewis CE, Kaplan SH, Davidson MB. Peer review by criteria mapping: criteria for diabetes mellitus. The use of decision-making in chart audit. Ann Intern Med 1975;83(6):761–770.

Grimm RH Jr, Shimoni K, Harlan WR Jr, Estes EH Jr. Evaluation of patient care protocol use by various providers. N Engl J Med 1975;292:507–511.

Grimshaw J, Russell IT. Achieving health gain through clinical guidelines. I: Developing scientifically valid guidelines. Quality in Health Care 1993;2:243–248.

Grimshaw JM, Russell IT. Effect of clinical guidelines on medical practice: a systematic review of rigorous evaluations. Lancet 1993;342:1317–1322.

Grimshaw JM, Russell IT. Acheiving health gain with clinical guidelines. II - Ensuring that guidelines change medical practice. Quality in Health Care 1994;3:45–52.

Grol R. National standard setting for quality of care in general practice: attitudes of general practitioners and resonse to a set of standards. Br J Gen Pract 1990;40:361–364.

Grol R. Implementing guidelines in general practice care. Quality in Health Care 1992;1:184–191.

Grol R. Development of guidelines for general practice care. Br J Gen Pract 1993;43:146–151.

Haine A, Feder G. Guidance on guidelines - Writing them is easier than making them work. Br Med J 1992;305:785–786.

Haines A, Jones R. Implementing findings of research. Br Med J 1994;308:1488–1493.

Hayward RS, Laupacis A. Initiating, conducting and maintaining guidelines development programs. Can Med Assoc J 1993;148(4):507–512.

Hayward RSA, Wilson MC, Tunis SR, Bass EB, Rubin HR, Hayes RB. More informative abstracts of articles describing clinical practice guidelines. Ann Intern Med 1993;118:731–737.

Heckerman DE, Nathwani BN. Toward normative expert systems: Part II. Probability-based representations for efficient knowledge acquisition and inference. Methods Inf Med 1992;31(2):106–116.

Herskovits EH, Cooper GF. Algorithms for Bayesian belief-network precomputation. Methods Inf Med 1991;30(2):81–89.

Hickam DH, Shortliffe EH, Bischoff MB, Scott AC, Jacobs CD. The treatment advice of a computer-based cancer chemotherapy protocol advisor. Ann Intern Med 1985;103(6):928–936.

Hofman PA. Critical path method: An important tool for co-ordinating clinical care. Journal on Quality Improvement 1993;19(7):235–246.

Hogg W. The role of computers in preventive medicine in a rural family practice. Can Med Assoc J 1990;143(1):33–37.

Hong Lam S. Implementation and evaluation of practice guidelines. Proc Annu Symp Comput Appl Med Care 1993:253–257.

Janson-Bjerklie S. Assessment and management of adults with asthma: guidelines for nurse practitioners. Nurse Practitioner Forum 1993;4(1):23–29.

Kamae IR, Greenes RA. A computational model of approximate Bayesian inference for associating clinical algorithms with decision analyses. Proc Annu Symp Comput Appl Med Care 1991:691–695.

Kaplan SH, Greenfield S. Criteria mapping: using logic in evaluation of processes of care. QRB Qual Rev Bull 1978;4(1):3–7.

Kassirer JP. Diagnostic Reasoning. Ann Intern Med 1989;110:893–900.

Kent DL, Shortliffe EH, Carlson RW, Bischoff MB, Jacobs CD. Improvements in data collection through physician use of a computer-based chemotherapy treatment consultant. J Clin Oncol 1985;3(10):1409–1417.

Komaroff AL. Algorithms and the 'Art of Medicine'. Am J Public Health 1982;72:10–12.

Komaroff HL, Flatley M, Browne C, Sherman H, Fineberg E, Knapp R. Quality, efficiency and cost of a physician-assistant protocol system for management of diabetes and hypertension. Diabetes 1976;25:297–306.

Kuipiers BJ, Kassirer JP. Causal reasoning in medicine: analysis of a protocol. Cogn Science 1984;8:363–385.

Lamas GA, Pfeffer MA, Hamm P, Wertheimer J, Rouleau JL, Braunwald E. Do the results of randomized clinical trials of cardiovascular drugs influence medical practice? The SAVE Investigators. N Engl J Med 1992;327(4):241–247.

Landgren FT, Harvey KJ, Mashford L, et al. Changing antibiotic prescribing by educational marketing. The Medical Journal of Australia 1988;149:595–599.

Lanzola G, Stefanelli M. Neoamemia: A knowledge-based system emulating diagnostic reasoning. Comput Biomed Res 1990;23:560–582.

Lichtenstein Michael J, Mulrow Cynthia D, Elwood Peter C. Guidelines for reading case-control studies. J Chronic Dis 1987;40:893–903.

Lilford RJ, Kelly M, Baines A, Cameron S, Cave M, Gutherie K, et al. Effect of using protocols on medical care: randomised trial of three methods of taking an antenatal history. Br Med J 1992;305:1181–1184.

Linnarsson R, Malmberg BG. Computerised medical record - a tool for quality assurance in primary health care. In: Lecture notes in medical informatics No.40 MIE90. (Eds: O'Moore,R; Bengtsson,S; Bryant,JR; Bryden,JS) Springer-Verlag, Berlin. 1990. pp. 693–695.

Lomas J. Words without action ? The production, dissemination and impact of concensus recommendations. Am Rev Publ Health 1991;12:41–65.

Lomas J. Making Clinical Policy Explicit - Legislative Policy Making and Lessons for Developing Practice Guidelines. Int J Technol Assess Health Care 1993;9:1:11–25.

Lomas J, Anderson GM, Domnick-Pierre K, Vayda E, Enkin MW, Hannah WJ. Do practice guidelines guide practice ? The effect of a consensus statement on the practice of physcians. N Engl J Med 1989;321:1311–1315.

Lomas J, Enkin M, Anderson GM, Hannah WJ, Vayda E, Singer J. Opinion leaders vs audit and feedback to implement practice guidelines. Delivery after previous caesarian section. JAMA 1991;265:2202–2207.

Lomas J, Haynes RB. A Taxonomy and Critical Review of Tested Strategies for the Applicaiton of Clinical Practice Recommendations: From "Official" to "Individual" Clinical Policy. Am J Prev Med 1987;4:77–94.

Lumsdon K. Pioneering protocols. Hospitals test the computer's use in patient care decisions. Hospitals 1993;67(9):18–21.

Margolis CZ. Uses of clinical algorithms. JAMA 1983;249:627.

Margolis Carmi Z, Cook Charles D, Adler Arlene, Geertsma Alex. Clinical Algorithms Teach Pediatric Decisionmaking More Effectively than Prose. Medical Care 1989;27(6):576–592.

Margolis CZ, Warshawsky S, Goldman L, Dagan O, Wirtschafter D. Effect of a computerised clinical algorith system on patient care. In: MEDINFO 89. (Eds: Barber,B; Cao,D; Qin,D; Wagner,G) North Holland Publ Comp, Amsterdam. 1989. 161–164.

Margolis CZ, Warshawsky SS, Goldman L, Dagan O, Wirtschafter D, Pliskin JS. Computerized algorithms and pediatricians' management of common problems in a community clinic. Acad Med 1992;67(4):282–284.

McAlister NH, Covvey DH, Tong C, Lee A, Wigle ED. Randomised controlled trial of computer assisted management of hypertension in primary care. Br Med J 1986;293:670–674.

McDonald CJ. Protocol-based computer reminders, the quality of care and the non-perfectability of man. N Engl J Med 1976;295(24):1351–1355.

McDonald C. Use of a computer to detect and respond to clinical events: Its effect on clinician behavior. Ann Intern Med 1976;84:162–167.

McDonald CJ, Hui SL, Smith DM, Tierney WM, Cohen SJ, Weinberger M, McCabe GP. Reminders to Physicians from an Introspective Computer Medical Record: A Two-Year Randomised Trial. Ann Intern Med 1984;100:130–138.

McDonald CJ, Hui SL, Tierney WM. Effects of computer reminders for influenza vaccination on morbidity during influenza epidemics. MD Comput 1992;9(5):304–312.

McDonald CJ, Wilson GA, McCabe GP. Physician responses to computer reminders. JAMA 1980;244(14):1579–1581.

Michelson S, Ben-Bassat M, MacNeil A, Weil MH. Computer implementation of hierachical modular approach to treament protocols. Methods Inf Med 1982;21:117–126.

Mittman BS, Tonesk X, Jacobson PD. Implementing Clinical Practice Guidelines: Social Influence Strategies and Practitioner Behaviour Change. QRB Qual Rev Bull 1992;18(12):413–422.

Morgan M, Studney DR, Barnett GO, Winickoff RN. Computerized concurrent review of prenatal care. QRB Qual Rev Bull 1978;4:33–36.

Murrey KO, Gottlieb LK, Schoenbaum SC. Implementing clinical guidelines: a quality management approach to reminder systems. QRB Qual Rev Bull 1992;18(12):423–433.

Oakeshott P, Kerry SM, Williams JE. Randomized controlled trial of the effect of the Royal College pf Radiologists' guidelines on general practioners' referrals for radiographic examination. Br J Gen Pract 1994;44:197–200.

Ogilvie-Harris DJ, Botsford DJ, Worden Hawker R. Elderly Patients with Hip Fractures: Improved Outcome with the Use of Care Maps with High-Quality Medical and Nursing Protocols. Journal of Orthopaedic Trauma 1993;7, No. 5:428–437.

O'Malley K, O'Brien E. Where are the guidelines for treating hypertension in elderly patients? Br Med J 1992;305:845–846.

Ornstein SM, Garr DR, Jenkins RG, Rust PF, Arnon A. Computer-generated physician and patient reminders. Tools to improve population adherence to selected preventive services. J Fam Pract 1991;32(1):82–90.

Osman LM, Abdalla MI, Beattie AG, Ross SJ, Russell IT, Friend JA, Legge JS, Douglas JG, Grampian Asthma Study of Integrated Care (GRASSIC). Reducing hospital admission through computer supported education for asthma patients. Br Med J 1994;308:568–571.

Oxman AD. Coordination of guidelines development. Can Med Assoc J 1993;148(8):1285–1288.

Pearson SD, Margolis CZ, Davis S, Schreier LK, Gottlieb LK. The clinical algorithm nosolgy: A method for comparing algorithmic guidelines. Med Decis Making 1992;12:123–131.

Petrucci K, Petrucci P, Canfield K, McComick KA, Kjerulff K, Parks P. Evaluation of UNIS: Urological Nursing Information System. Proc Annu Symp Comput Appl Med Care 1991;:43–47.

Petryshen PR, Petryshen PM. The case management model: an innovative approach to the delivery of patient care. J Adv Nurs 1992;17:1188–1194.

Pringle M. The new agenda for general practice computing [editorial]. Br Med J 1990;301(6756):827–828.

Purves IN, Cowley C, Bainbridge M, Grimshaw JM. Using guidlines (letter). Br Med J 1992;305:1364.

Purves IN, Grimshaw JM. Computer generated protocols (letter). Br Med J 1993;306:460.

Randall T, Muir J, Mant D. Choosing the preventive workload in general practice: practical application of the Coronary Prevention Group guidelines and Dundee coronary risk-disk. Br Med J 1992;305(6847):227–231.

Rucker DW, Maron DJ, Shortliffe EH. Temporal representation of clinical algorithms using expert-system and database tools. Comput Biomed Res 1990;23(3):222–239.

Rucker DW, Shortliffe EH. A methodology for implementing clinical algorithms using expert-system and database tools. Proc Annu Symp Comput Appl Med Care 1989:33–37.

Russell IT, Grimshaw JM. The effectiveness of referral guidelines: a review of the methods and findings of published evaluations. In: Hospital Referrals. (Eds: Roland,M; Coulter,A) Oxford University Press, Oxford. 1992. .

Sackett DL. Rules of evidence and clinical recommendations on the use of antithrombotic agents. Chest 1986;86(2, Suppl.):2S–3S.

Sackett DL. Rules of evidence and clinical recommendations for the management of patients. Canadian Journal of Cardiology 1993;9(6):487–489.

Schoenbaum SC, Gottlieb LK. Algorithm based improvement of clinical quality. Br Med J 1990;301:1374–1376.

Sever P, Beevers G, Bulpitt C, Lever A, Ramsay L, Reid J, Swales J. Management guidelines in essential hypertension: report of the second working party of the British Hypertension Society. Br Med J 1993;306:983–987.

Sheldon TA. Changing the measure of quality in the NHS: from purchasing activity to purchasing protocols. Quality in Health Care 1993;2:149–150.

Shiffman RN, Greenes RA. Use of augmented decision table to convert probabilistic data into clinical algorithms for the diagnosis of appendicitis. Proc Annu Symp Comput Appl Med Care 1991:686–690.

Shiffman RN, Greenes RA. Rule set reduction using augmented decision table and semantic subsumption techniques: application to cholesterol guidelines. Proc Annu Symp Comput Appl Med Care 1992:339–343.

Shiffman RN, Leape LL, Greenes RA. Translation of appropriateness criteria into practice guidelines: Application of decision table techniques to the RAND criteria for coronary artery bypass graft. Proc Annu Symp Comput Appl Med Care 1993:248–252.

Society for Medical Decision Making Committee on Standardization of Clinical Algorithms. Proposal for Clinical Algorithm Standards. Med Decis Making 1992;12:149–154.

Somerville MA. Ethics and clinical practice guidelines. Can Med Assoc J 1993;148(7):1133–1137.

Sommers LS, Scholtz R, Shepherd RM, Starkweather DB. Physician involvement in quality assurance. Medical Care 1984;22:1115–1138.

Sox HC, Sox CH, Tompkins RK. The training of physcians' assistants: The use of a clinical algorithm system. N Engl J Med 1973;288:818–824.

Sox HC Jr, Woolf SH. Evidence-based practice guidelines from the US Preventive Services Task Force [editorial; comment]. JAMA 1993;269(20):2678.

Tape TG, Stoupa RA, Campbell JR. Implementing guidelines in ambulatory practice. Proc Annu Symp Comput Appl Med Care 1992:806–807.

Thomas JC, Moore A, Qualls PE. The effect on cost of medical care for patients treated with an automated clinical audit system. Journal of Medical Systems 1983;7:307–313.

Thomas Siewert. Standard setting in the Netherlands: impact of the human factor on guideline development. Br J Gen Pract 1994;June 1994:242–243.

Tierney WM, Hui SL, McDonald CJ. Delayed feedback of physician performance versus immediate reminders to perform preventive care. Effects on physician compliance. Med Care 1986;24(8):659–666.

Tierney WM, McDonald CJ, Martin DK, Rogers MP. Computerized display of past test results. Effect on outpatient testing. Ann Intern Med 1987;107(4):569–574.

Tierney WM, Miller ME, Overhage JM, McDonald CJ. Physician inpatient order writing on microcomputer workstations. Effects on resource utilization. JAMA 1993;269(3):379–383.

Unstable angina guideline panel (Ed.). Unstable angina: Diagnosis and management. (94–0602) (Clinical Practice Guideline.) Agency for Health Care Policy and Research Publications, Rockville, MD. 1994.

van der Lei J, Musen MA, van der Does E, Man in't Veld AJ, van Bemmel JH. Comparison of computer-aided and human review of general practitioners' management of hypertension. Lancet 1991;338(8781):1504–1508.

van Duijn NP, Brouwer HJ, Lamberts H. Use of symptoms and signs to diagnose maxillary sinusitis in general practice: comparison with ultrasonography . Br Med J 1992;305(6855):684–687.

Veingarten MA, Bazal D, Shannon HS. Computerised protocol for preventative medicine: A controlled self audit in Family Practice. Fam Pract 1989;6:120–124.

Walton JD, Musen MA, Combs DM, Lane CD, Shortliffe EH, Fagan LM. Graphical access to medical expert systems: III. Design of a knowledge acquisition environment. Methods Inf Med 1987;26(3):78–88.

Weingarten MA, Bazel D, Shannon H. Computerised protocol for preventative medicine: A controlled self-audit in family practice. Fam Pract 1989;6(2):120–124.

White LJ, Ball JR. The clinical efficacy assessment project of the American College of Physicians. Int J Technol Assess Health Care 1985;1:169–174.

Wimberley Edward T, Blazyk Stan. Monitoring Patient Outcome Following Discharge: A Computerized Geriatric Case-Management System. Health and Social Work 1989;November 1989:269–276.

Wirtschafter D, Carpenter JT, Mesel E. A consultant-extender system for breast cancer adjuvant chemotherapy. Ann Intern Med 1979;90:396–401.

Wirtschafter D, Summers J, Jackson JR, Brooks CM, Turner M. Continuing medical educaiton using algorithms: a controlled trial assessment of effect of neonatal care. American Journal of Diseases of Childhood 1986;140:791–797.

Woolf SH. Practice guidelines: a new reality in medicine. I. Recent developments. Arch Intern Med 1990;150(9):1811–1818.

Woolf SH. The process of developing practice guidelines. Decubitus 1991;4(2):28–31.

Woolf SH. Practice Guidelines, a New Reality in Medicine: Methods of Developing Guidelines. Arch Intern Med 1992;152:946–952.

Woolf SH. Practice guidelines: a new reality in medicine. III. Impact on patient care. Arch Intern Med 1993;153(23):2646–2655.

Woolf SH, Battista RN, Anderson GM, Logan AG, Wang E. Assessing the Clinical Effectiveness of Preventive Maneuvers:Analytic Principles and Systematic Methods in Reviewing Evidence and Developing Clinical Practice Recommendations.   A Report by the Canadian Task Force on the Periodic Health Examination. J Clin Epidemiol 1990;43(9):891–905.

Zander K. Critical pathways. Chap. 9. In: Total Quality Management: The Health Care Pioneers. (Eds: Melum,MM; Sinior,MK) American Hospital Publishing. 1992. 305–314.

AUTHOR INDEX